Using Technology in Human Services Education: Going the Distance

Using Technology in Human Services Education: Going the Distance has been co-published simultaneously as *Journal of Technology in Human Services,* Volume 18, Numbers 1/2 2001.

Using Technology in Human Services Education: Going the Distance

Goutham M. Menon, PhD
Nancy K. Brown, PhD
Editors

Using Technology in Human Services Education: Going the Distance has been co-published simultaneously as *Journal of Technology in Human Services*, Volume 18, Numbers 1/2,2001.

Routledge
Taylor & Francis Group
NEW YORK AND LONDON

Using Technology in Human Services Education: Going the Distance has been co-published simultaneously as *Journal of Technology in Human Services*™, Volume 18, Numbers 1/2 2001.

First published 2001 by
The Haworth Press, Inc., 10 Alice Street, Binghamton, NY 13904-1580

This edition published 2013 by Routledge
711 Third Avenue, New York, NY 10017, USA
2 Park Square, Milton Park, Abingdon, Oxon OX14 4RN

First issued in hardback 2017

Routledge is an imprint of the Taylor & Francis Group, an informa business

Cover design by Thomas J. Mayshock Jr.

Library of Congress Cataloging-in-Publication Data

Using technology in human services education : going the distance / Goutham M. Menon, Nancy K. Brown, editors.
p. cm.
Includes bibliographical references and index.
ISBN 0-7890-1371-1 (alk. paper)–ISBN 0-7890-1372-X (pbk. : alk. paper)
1. Social work education–United States. 2. Educational technology–United States I. Menon, Goutham M. II. Brown, Nancy K.

HV11.U77 2001
361.3′07′1073–dc21 2001046327

ISBN 13: 978-0-7890-1372-9 (pbk)
ISBN 13: 978-1-1384-6178-9 (hbk)

ABOUT THE EDITORS

Goutham M. Menon, PhD, is Assistant Professor at the College of Social Work, University of South Carolina. He completed the Master's degree in Social Work from the Madras School of Social Work, India, and the doctoral degree from the School of Social Work, University of Illinois at Urbana-Champaign. Dr. Menon's area of work is focused on the utilization of technology for Social Work practice and education. He is particularly interested in drawing up standards of practice for online, web-based counseling services and has presented papers in this area in national conferences. He also looks at issues stemming from online support groups, electronic advocacy, and has a deep interest in developing necessary tools for the ethical utilization of the Internet for research.

Dr. Menon is on the board of editors for the *Journal of Technology in Human Services* and also reviews papers for the journal *Social Development Issues*. He manages the websites for the Inter-University Consortium for International Social Development, the International Commission of the Council on Social Work Education and oversees the working of SWAN. Dr. Menon also follows developments in the areas of International Social Development, Immigration Policy and Asian Mental Health.

Nancy K. Brown, PhD, is Assistant Professor at the College of Social Work, University of South Carolina. She completed her master's degree in social work and her doctorate at the University at Albany, in New York. Dr. Brown has worked primarily in the area of women and addictions. She has explored the recovery process in women, and its association with high-risk behavior in recovery from crack-cocaine addiction. Her current research examines parental self-efficacy in substance abuse prevention. Her research methodology includes qualitative methods as well as a web-based online survey. She is interested in exploring the comparison between web-based research and traditional qualitative methods.

Dr. Brown became interested in technology after coming to the University of South Carolina. Her research in this area has explored student characteristics and their association with the adaptation to and adoption of technology.

Using Technology in Human Services Education: Going the Distance

CONTENTS

Going the Distance: Using Technology in Human Services Education

Nancy K. Brown
Goutham M. Menon

One day in the fall of 1961, at St. Mary's Grammar School in Rahway, New Jersey, Sr. Martina rolled a television into the classroom right before lunchtime. The students had heard rumors about this upcoming event, and here was proof that modern times had materialized. If Educational TV could enter the pedagogically rigid halls of St. Mary's, could the discovery of life on Mars lag far behind? What they learned in the following weeks was that "Educational TV," the prototype of modern Distance Education, was not exactly what the title led them to expect.

Those students learned a few Spanish words, and conjugated a few sentences. But mostly, they found that educational television amounted to little more than a time-filler during slow periods. Occasionally they watched special events. The Mercury space program was in full tilt, and they watched the Mercury-Atlas rocket launches, perhaps inspiring some of those young men and women to dream of careers in science.

Distance Education, or "Educational TV" as it was known back then, made its debut in a less than astounding fashion. However, that

Nancy K. Brown is Assistant Professor, and Goutham M. Menon is Assistant Professor, College of Social Work, University of South Carolina, Columbia, SC 29208.

[Haworth co-indexing entry note]: "Going the Distance: Using Technology in Human Services Education." Brown, Nancy K., and Goutham M. Menon. Co-published simultaneously in *Journal of Technology in Human Services* (The Haworth Press, Inc.) Vol. 18, No. 1/2, 2001, pp. 1-4; and: *Using Technology in Human Services Education: Going the Distance* (ed: Goutham M. Menon, and Nancy K. Brown) The Haworth Press, Inc., 2001, pp. 1-4. Single or multiple copies of this article are available for a fee from The Haworth Document Delivery Service [1-800-342-9678, 9:00 a.m. - 5:00 p.m. (EST). E-mail address: getinfo@haworthpressinc.com].

school, a little non-innovative, small town school, foresaw the potential power of this tool enough to invest in it and bring this technology into the classroom. The difficulty in establishing the thoughtful integration of technology into the traditional classroom remains our struggle today. The technology is often way ahead of us, and we are constantly striving to catch up to it. Finding ways to maximize the potential of distance education, which is now infused with the formidable power of the World Wide Web, is our challenge. Ultimately, we have to see that distance learning is only slightly more than tangentially related to technology; it is ultimately and precisely about education. As we get more accustomed to the thrills of a millennia of technological advances, the tail will stop wagging the dog, and we will work hard to ensure that what we do is "best practices" in education, just as we would in the field through critique, evaluation, and research.

Currently, the majority of higher education institutions in the United States has begun distance education programs. The United States Department of Education reported that as of 1995, about 25% of all institutions of higher learning offered complete degree programs through distance education courses, and this number is rapidly growing (Matthews, 1999). According to technology research conducted by the International Data Corporation, 2.2 million college students will be enrolled in distance-learning courses within two years (IDC, 1999).

The implementation of distance education programs has gathered momentum. But, unlike the development of the underlying technology (i.e., the computer chip, the PC, and even the Internet itself), the evolution of distance education is not occurring as a monumental event, but rather as a force that is driven by the inexorable need to bring the goods to market, i.e., the learning to the students. Still, it is evolving at an extraordinary pace.

The University of South Carolina continues to host a weeklong conference on the use of technology in education and practice in the field of social work and other human services. This special edition represents a selection of papers chosen for their capacity to provide useful information to both practitioners and educators. The issue begins with Rebecca Ashery's discussion of the current status of technology utilization in graduate schools of social work. From her work emerge a number of themes and recommendations for schools that vie for leadership in the field of human services and technology.

When a school utilizes distance learning technology to merge resources with another school, a blending of cultures takes place between the two schools. Each school has a unique perspective, but as Priscilla R. Smith and Nikki W. Wingerson point out, there must emerge from this union a new culture that operates to benefit the learners equally at both locations. The means to successfully creating the new culture may lie in increased interaction, particularly face-to-face contact between both sites.

John J. Newhouse reminds us that distance education has changed continuously over the last 30 years, and that strategies for teaching in these new media must also adapt. In his paper, he provides the reader with a framework from which to design distance learning courses that fully utilize the unique environments these courses offer. He offers an integration of instructional approaches typically found in the traditional platform classroom (e.g., presentations, discussions, group work, and role plays) into these settings.

Aside from the overall structure and design of distance education courses in general, Marie Huff considers the impact of technological tools in teaching specific course content, in this case, diversity. She reports on the positive experience students had when they utilized e-mail and electronic discussion groups as part of the instructional milieu on human services courses in diversity.

Perhaps the most difficult and controversial content to be taught via distance learning is practice-related skill. Janet Pray looks at the development of the essential practice skills of critical thinking, theory application, ethical decision-making, and achieving a professional identity. Dr. Pray shows us how discussion forums can increase students' depth of thinking about these issues.

Christine B. Hagan, Marilyn K. Potts, and John Oliver show how a Site Advisory Committee (SAC) can increase students' socialization into the profession. They report on a particular SAC that succeeded in creating a reference group for off-campus students by providing a strong linkage between the university, the host site and the local community. They include recommendations for creating successful SACs for off-campus settings.

When schools of social work and human services programs implement distance learning programs, evaluation is essential in determining the success of these programs. These evaluations lead to interesting questions, as C. David Hollister and Youngmin Kim point out. What increased students' learning in interactive television courses? How do students need to be supported in order to feel connected to the program? Do graduates from these types of programs adopt more electronic technology into their practice? Their results report satisfaction with these courses as equal to or higher than traditional program graduates.

Human service professionals know that learning is a lifelong endeavor. In practice, the professional requires access to state-of-the-art information, and the delivery of technology-supported training in their local communities. Philip M. Ouellette and Scott Sells describe the collaboration between two universities to create a dynamic learning telelearning community to train practitioners working with troubled youth and families. Their work helps us to understand what conditions "facilitate or hinder learning efficacy" in the collaborative environment.

Ultimately, those who complete programs in human services become professionals in many practice contexts. Experience gained in the educational setting may increase practitioners' use of technology in the field. As Kunkel and Yowell demonstrate, welfare and workforce reforms are creating new challenges for individual agencies to provide services to this population. Technological tools can be employed to facilitate case management through collaborative strategies. Kunkel and Yowell share information that is useful in negotiating the transition toward Collaborative Case Management.

Another example of how technological tools can help in the learning process is exemplified by the work of Robert Watkins where he describes the use of Geographic Information Systems to identify and meet information needs of their field placement agency.

And, finally, Julie Miller-Cribbs' work helps us to keep in our vision the fact that the gap is increasing between individuals who have access to technology and those who do not. She explores the effect of this growing problem on the clients that many human service professionals deal with, and points out strategies for minimizing issues regarding the inequality of access.

REFERENCES

International Data Corporation. (1999). College Distance Learning to Triple by 2002. *Technical Training*, July-August, v. 10, i4, p3.

Matthews, D. (1999). The origins of distance education and its use in the United States. *Technological Horizons in Education*, Sept., v. 27, i2.

The Utilization of Technology in Graduate Schools of Social Work

Rebecca Sager Ashery

SUMMARY. Fifteen faculty from graduate schools of social work and staff from three social work organizations were interviewed by telephone for this qualitative study to describe utilization of technology. Schools were engaged in technology activities that ranged from basic to special technology projects. For the most part there was unevenness in the use of technology within each school and between schools. A number of themes emerged. Eleven recommendations are given to help schools to become leaders in the field of social work and technology. *[Article copies available for a fee from The Haworth Document Delivery Service: 1-800-342-9678. E-mail address: <getinfo@haworthpressinc.com> Website: <http://www.HaworthPress.com> © 2001 by The Haworth Press, Inc. All rights reserved.]*

KEYWORDS. Technology utilization, schools of social work

Social workers enter the profession because they are extroverted "people-persons" who enjoy interaction and communication with others. They often shy away from words like "research" because that puts people into a "guinea pig" category of testing, numbers and data. Likewise there is a tendency to be suspicious of computers that will also come between them and human contact with those in need. How-

Rebecca Sager Ashery, DSW, is affiliated with the Substance Abuse and Mental Health Services Administration, Center for Substance Abuse Prevention.

[Haworth co-indexing entry note]: "The Utilization of Technology in Graduate Schools of Social Work." Ashery, Rebecca Sager. Co-published simultaneously in *Journal of Technology in Human Services* (The Haworth Press, Inc.) Vol. 18, No. 1/2, 2001, pp. 5-18; and: *Using Technology in Human Services Education: Going the Distance* (ed: Goutham M. Menon, and Nancy K. Brown) The Haworth Press, Inc., 2001, pp. 5-18. Single or multiple copies of this article are available for a fee from The Haworth Document Delivery Service [1-800-342-9678, 9:00 a.m. - 5:00 p.m. (EST). E-mail address: getinfo@haworthpressinc.com].

ever, social workers now find themselves in a digital economy that poses challenges to the profession. There are new demands from health and social service agencies for more cost control, outcome measures, quality performance and information technology. Whether social workers like it or not, they must enter the digital age.

A search on the Internet is paradoxical to the above paragraph. The Internet is brimming with information on the use of technology in human services and in social work. There is a Technology Conference for Social Work Education and Practice now in its third year sponsored by the University of South Carolina College of Social Work. There are two journals on technology in human services: *Journal of Technology in Human Services* and *New Technology in the Human Services*, a number of social work and technology courses (Social Work 211-no date; Information Technology and Social Work-no date), books on social work and/or human services and technology (Schwartz, 1984; Mizrahi, Downing, Fasano, Friedland, McCullough, and Shapiro, 1991; Karger and Levine, 1999), clinical software that has been developed for use to assist and/or educate clients (Cahill, 1994; Software Review Form, 1997; FamilyWorks-no date), informational databases, and Online discussion forums for social workers (World Wide Web Resources for Social Work, 2000; Social Work Access Network, 1997). Many of the universities have developed distance education social work courses, however, it should be noted that the definition of "distance education" varies among schools. International information on social work and technology in other countries can be found on the Internet.

The use of computers for research purposes has long been established. Now, however, instead of a mainframe, students and researchers are able to utilize qualitative and quantitative software packages at their desktops. The use of technology for databases for clients and other information sometimes makes social workers arch their backs in alarm regarding issues of confidentiality and privacy. Computer matching for welfare fraud, while having some good points, also makes one consider the consequences of privacy invasion. The use of software for clinical practice has been demonstrated to be effective and useful, unfortunately, there has been little use made of it. In some preliminary discussions with people in the field, it appears that there is a "disconnect" between the technology available in human services and the audience of social workers. One expert estimated that only

5-10% of the social workers use the information on the web or use technology at their work except for e-mail and word processing.

With the demands of the digital age, the question arises regarding what graduate schools of social work are doing to prepare students in technology. Are graduate schools leaders in the field or is the field leading them? There is very little specific information regarding the use of technology in graduate schools. All schools appear to have a website. One can get some hints of technology utilization by the layout and extensiveness of the web site, but it is difficult to obtain a total picture.

There is a recognition that the traditional "classroom" is changing via technology (Reck, no date). Are schools utilizing technology extensively? Are they keeping up with the demands of the field? How will schools be utilizing the new high speed Internet2 as it enters onto their campus? Is there a potential for graduate schools of social work to become technological "haves" and "have-nots"?

In order to learn more about the use of technology in graduate schools of social work, it was decided to contact a minimum of 10 schools to find out about technology utilization. It should be noted that the original study plan was to focus only on the utilization of Internet2 (Abilene Project) by graduate schools of social work. However, after six preliminary calls, it turned out that the schools currently were not involved in Internet2 even though their universities were Internet2 partners. It appeared that the schools were waiting for word from their university rather than being proactively involved. Therefore, the subject shifted to the use of technology in general including Internet2.

TARGET GROUP

As a selection device, it was decided to interview schools whose universities were Internet2 partners since questions regarding Internet2 participation were planned. Twenty-six deans were contacted by e-mail. There was an attempt to have geographic distribution and small and large schools. A list of graduate schools was obtained on the web from the Council on Social Work Education (CSWE) website. The e-mail addresses were obtained from the social work web page at each school. (The university web page was contacted first, which was linked to the school of social work). The e-mail explained the study and asked the deans to name the person (with the phone number) on their faculty who was the most knowledgeable regarding technology. The e-mail specified faculty rather than a "computer-tech" person. Eighteen responses were received and faculty from fourteen graduate schools were interviewed. One MSW candidate school that had a BSW program was interviewed to make a total of fifteen schools interviewed. In addition, several social work organizations were interviewed as well as individuals known to the field.

SEMI-STRUCTURED INTERVIEW GUIDE

A semi-structured interview guide was used in a phone conversation that took from 20 minutes to 45 minutes depending on how much the respondent had to say about technology activities. The guide focused on the type of technology used in the school and how it was being used. Questions were asked about web pages, CD-ROMs, videoconferencing, etc. Faculty were also asked about collaborative activities, participation on a technology task force/committee through the university or school, training for faculty and students, plans to use Internet2, issues and problems in using technology, and what they saw as the future for social work in technology.

FINDINGS

Since this was a qualitative study with only fifteen schools of social work interviewed and several organizations, the findings will be reported by emerging themes that arose during the discussions. Although the numbers are small, from the discussions, these themes appear to be reliable and could be applicable to the field.

Overarching Themes

Schools were engaged in technology activities that ranged from basic to special technology project(s). Even those schools that did not have the latest equipment might be engaged in an innovative activity that a more "wired" school was not engaged in. For example, several schools that had more resources had made a conscious decision not to get involved in distance education.

There were several overarching themes that emerged: (1) All schools of social work were involved to some degree in the use of technology; (2) Most schools had not developed a comprehensive plan for the utilization of technology; (3) There was an unevenness in the use of technology within each school and between schools; In most schools the technology was driven by the interests of less than a handful of faculty; (4) Much depended on the leadership within the University and the leadership of the dean in the school of social work; and (5) There was concern regarding the obsolescence of technology and technology funding.

1. Use of Technology. All schools of social work were involved in varying aspects of technology. All had computer labs either within the university or within the school itself. For the most part, these labs were used for training in computer skills, web searches and research. All schools had some kind of training in computers for students and faculty. Research students were using qualitative and quantitative software packages via desktop computers. All schools had a web page, but not all faculties had web pages. In some cases the university was requiring that all faculty have web pages. Some faculty (varied within and between schools) put their syllabus and additional class information on the web. All faculty used e-mail, word processing and some were using Power Point. All schools had connections via the computer to the library. Some schools were videotaping student interviews with clients. Videotaping interviews has been used as a teaching tool for many years. Several schools had a course in social work and technology. Most of these courses focused on developing web-based skills. Professors utilized technology (Internet, software) most often for policy and research courses. Since policy changes so frequently, the use of the web was seen as essential for this course. Several schools had conducted a forum or panel discussion via satellite. One school had used video-conferencing and another stated that video-conferencing was "on the way." One professor had developed software on how to conduct an interview. This professor had also developed a multimedia test for the supervisor exam for worker safety in child welfare. No one else interviewed had engaged in software development. The use of technology for clinical practice has lagged behind other areas, mainly because of the "in-person" issues.

Many schools were engaged in some form of distance education with a branch or branches of the university located away from the main campus. This consisted of either one-way video and two-way audio or two-way audio and video. All schools engaged in distance education had assistants located at the remote sites. One school was starting an experimental distance education program with information on the web, videotapes of lectures sent to students and a one time face-to-face meeting with the professor. There was no school that had distance education courses completely on the web like the George Washington University Education Technology Leadership program.

2. *Comprehensive Plan.* Only a few schools stated that they had some type of comprehensive plan for the use of technology. Many schools developed plans for the implementation of specific technology (e.g., distance education). Most plans were "piecemeal" and there did not appear to be an overall comprehensive plan to integrate technology into the curriculum. A plan should include a vision statement, goals, objectives, implementation, action steps, and follow-up evaluation.

For the past three years the University of Maryland School of Social Work has used a strategic planning process to develop and implement technology. The strategic planning effort started with conducting a needs assessment of the faculty, administrators and students regarding their use of technology. The needs assessment included surveys and qualitative interviews regarding access to computers, how they are used (e-mail, statistical packages, etc.), identification of types of technology (audio, video) relied on in their everyday work, problems encountered, and training and technology needs. The needs assessment is conducted yearly, and the findings are used to prioritize the acquisition of hardware, software and the provision of training. Based on the findings, the strategic plan is modified yearly. For example, on the basis of findings, training was shifted to outside vendors rather than conducting training in-house. The yearly needs assessment helps the school to focus on the shifting needs of the audience.

3. *Faculty Knowledge.* An overriding theme was the need to have a "buy-in" from the entire faculty on using technology. Even the schools that were well "wired" reported an unevenness among the faculty regarding knowledge of and use of technology. Since the majority of social work programs are heavily clinical, it is difficult to help faculty see how technology could help in an area that depends on face-to-face contact. In many cases it appeared that there was only a handful of faculty within a school that were using the technology for their classes. And only one or two were actually using technology

innovatively, e.g., getting grants in technology, conducting studies in technology, active class use, etc. Many study participants mentioned that there was no overriding motivation for faculty since the use or development of technology is not linked to tenure. Universally, everyone interviewed mentioned the need to train faculty "one-on-one." Faculty learn better in a one-on-one situation and did not want to go to a class for training. Most schools either already had or were making arrangements for "on-call" direct tech support for faculty and direct one-on-one instruction. There was also mention of the "age" issue, with "younger" faculty perceived as more amenable and knowledgeable regarding technology than "older" faculty. Several mentioned the "shame" factor. For example, when one sees a colleague using Power Point, then there is pressure to learn and present with Power Point.

4. Leadership. It appeared from the conversations that it was important to have the leadership and support from "the top." A supportive university and a supportive dean were important. For example, one university had a Center for Innovation and Technology in Learning where faculty could go for help if they wanted to try new approaches. That same university also gave internal technology grants to encourage faculty innovation. Another university had software for making web pages with expectations that faculty in all colleges would use it as a template to develop their own individual web pages. Another university, which encouraged distance education, had a distance education department to help university faculty develop distance education courses. Underlying this supportive help was an issue of centralization and decentralization regarding technology within a university. Some universities appeared to have strong centralized support services while others were more decentralized with each school responsible for most aspects of technology. There are pros and cons to both approaches. Since this topic was not a major part of the study, I did not discuss the details of this issue with participants. This issue lends itself to a separate study.

5. Technology Obsolescence and Funding. Everyone mentioned equipment obsolescence and funding for technology as a major concern. There was a fear of buying expensive technology only to have it become obsolete in eighteen months. Everyone stated that technology was changing too rapidly to keep up. There were hopes that this rapidity would reach a plateau. However, there was also the reality of thinking in a new paradigm of eighteen months for equipment replacement.

LIST OF PROJECTS

Some schools were engaged in "special" projects and/or studies on technology. These projects indicate some creativity and testing of technology uses. They are worth mentioning to obtain a picture of the scope and variety of what the schools were doing. The projects are in various stages of planning and implementation. It should be noted that these types of projects might not be considered "special" uses of technology for other university departments, but for social work they are.

1. Faculty will develop a web page for each course with a hyperlink directly to the book or article. The student will never have to go to the library. *University of California-Berkeley*
2. A semi-virtual distance education PhD program in social work for current MSW faculty. There would be 8-10 students with supplemental visits by the professor. *University of Utah*
3. Research project-fall '99–Course Social Work and the Law will be taught (1) in person; (2) total asynchronously on the web; (3) combined. Comparisons between these methods and between other courses will be made. *Ohio University*
4. Software development and multimedia program for child welfare workers on safety has been developed. *University of Texas-Arlington*
5. School of Social Work is a member of a university committee working on the issue of submitting the final dissertation electronically. *University of Wisconsin-Madison*
6. Visual echo scan–One enters data on a client and it will tell you what is happening. Software templates will be developed for case materials or to assess human behavior. *Columbia University*
7. Agency descriptions will be on the web so students can select field placements. *Syracuse University*
8. School had an endowed institute with a technological focus, but no operational funds. *Florida State University*
9. Pilot project–There will be contacts to the student's field placement agency via the Internet. This will not replace in-person visits. *University of South Carolina*
10. Study–There will be a pre/post test of student technology skills: when they enter school, when they graduate. *University of South Carolina*

11. Working with curriculum committee to infuse technology into every course. *University of South Carolina, University of New Hampshire*
12. Host for 3rd annual Technology and Social Work Conference. *University of South Carolina*
13. Home-net–This is a special project to virtually link people who want to buy a house and have no credit to resources on the Web. They will be taught how to use a database and will have assistance in finding resources. *Case Western Reserve University*
14. Faculty is serving on a National Committee with the National Institute of Social Work in London to address quality standards for health information on the Internet in order to empower the user. *New York University*
15. A class contacted students on the Internet from Romania, then had face-to-face visit. *Case Western Reserve University*
16. World Wide Web Resources for Social Workers online with 30,500 links. Co-sponsored by New York University's Ehrenkranz School of Social Work and the Mount Sinai-NYU Medical Center & Health System.
17. Web course in a box–University developed a template for web based courses for use by all departments; 30% to 40% of all university classes have supplemental web sites using template. *Virginia Commonwealth University*

RECOMMENDATIONS

Given that graduate schools of social work need to be in the forefront of technology, the following recommendations are made:

1. Comprehensive Plan. Schools of social work should develop a vision statement and comprehensive strategic plan regarding the utilization of technology. Without a comprehensive plan, there is no overall program direction for technology in the school, inviting a "piecemeal" approach that encourages frustration and negativity. For example, the school should think about where they want to be technologically in the year 2005. Faculty should be actively involved in the development of this plan and should have "ownership" in the plan. It is most important that the entire faculty be on-board. The plan should be a five-year plan, with modifications at intervals during those five years based on new technology and findings. The need for equipment upgrades should be built into the plan. This comprehensive plan should also include a plan for implementation. This plan should include a decision on a basic level of technology knowledge for faculty and a level of integration of technology in the classroom and field placement.

2. *Committees.* There should be a standing Committee on Technology within the school. The technology committee would be involved in developing a technology plan. There may be subcommittees or ad hoc committees as appropriate. The school should strive to have as many faculty as possible participate. In addition, the school should be proactive in joining university based technology committees/task forces.

3. *Internet2.* At this point it appears that the schools of engineering and medicine are mainly involved in the launching of Internet2 (Abilene Project). Schools of social work should not wait for the university to invite them to participate. They should take a proactive stance in participating whenever possible on committees to gain a better understanding of Internet2, learn what the possibilities are for utilizing Internet2 and begin planning for that utilization. It did not appear that any of the schools of social work had a full grasp of the potential of Internet2.

4. *University Support.* Schools of social work need to take advantage of everything their university has to offer in the way of technology support, e.g., building web pages, helping with distance education, etc. It is also preferable, depending on the numbers of faculty, to have a technical staff person located within the school to "troubleshoot" when something goes wrong with hardware/software and to help teach faculty one-on-one.

5. *Joint Projects-Other Departments.* Schools of social work should develop joint projects using technology with other departments within the university such as nursing, criminology, psychology, etc. This is a good way to combine and stretch resources. In addition, the schools are taking risks together in terms of technological innovation.

6. *Tenure Rules.* Schools of social work should work with the university on changing the tenure rules to include technology. This may include the development and testing of software, which may take as long or longer than a general research project. It may also include setting up a distance education program and evaluating it. Because there is no "credit" for tenure, there is no motivation for faculty to become involved in technology.

7. Certificate of Technology in Human Services. Schools may think about offering a certificate program of Technology in Human Services. This certificate would be similar to certificates offered in clinical social work or in management for human services. This program may be directed to social workers working in public/private agencies who will use technology for training, database information, client assessment, client therapy, conferencing, etc. The purpose of this program would be to help social workers become knowledgeable about how technology can be utilized in the human services work world and to help them become leaders in technology in human services. The program would be similar to the George Washington University Education Technology Leadership (ETL) program.

8. Centers of Excellence. A minimum of four schools could collaborate to become a consortium or Centers of Excellence, offering students an array of lectures, programming, conferences, etc., via technology that each school could not offer alone. Establishing Centers of Excellence may bring in a larger student enrollment, bring in more grant awards, and save money in terms of resources.

9. Partnerships with Private Industry. Schools of social work should seek partnerships with private industry to help provide technological resources for the school and to work on joint projects. There are numerous projects that could be done ranging from technology access to poor communities, helping the poor to train and find jobs in technology, mentoring at risk kids in technology, etc. Social work has the access to vulnerable populations and the knowledge to work with these populations whereas private industry has the equipment and knowledge in technology.

10. Grant Applications. Schools of social work should apply for grant applications in technology. They could submit joint grant applications with other university departments, other schools of social work, community agencies, etc. In addition, when applying for a "regular" grant, schools of social work should incorporate technology into the grant. This will allow the school to "experiment" with technology and request the purchase of equipment.

11. Other Sources of Funding. Schools of social work should find new sources of funding for technology, such as collaboration with private industry and grants mentioned above. In addition, one may want to appeal to alumni, special gifts or endowments, look at new sources for grant money, contract money, etc. Schools need to be creative in thinking about funding for technology.

CONCLUSION

In summary there are both commonalities and variances regarding the use of technology by graduate schools of social work. Although this is a profession that is dominated by face-to-face interactions, it is quickly becoming evident that technology can be used in a variety of ways by graduate schools and by the profession in general. A number of issues and barriers exist; however, many study participants believe that the future for social work and technology is bright with endless creative possibilities. In addition, participants expressed the opinion that eventually technology would merge "seamlessly" as a vital part of the classroom and the profession. Participants expressed concern that the schools that did not keep up would be left behind.

REFERENCES

Cahill, J. (1994) Health works: Interactive AIDS education videogames. *Computers in Human Services*, *11*(1/2), 159-176.

FamilyWorks: *Parenting Wisely* (no date) Retrieved March 19, 2000 from the World Wide Web: http://www.familyworksinc.com/content.html

Information Technology and Social Work-Course Syllabus, SW 810 (no date) Dr. Jerry Finn University of New Hampshire, Retrieved March 19, 2000 from the World Wide Web: http://www.unh.edu/social-work/SW810/web.htm

Journal of Technology in Human Services. New York, The Haworth Press, Inc.

Karger, H.J., and Levine J. (1999) *The Internet and Technology for the Human Services*. Addison Wesley Longman, Inc. New York.

Mizrahi, T., Downing, J., Fasano, R., Friedland, P., McCullough, M., and Shapiro, J. (1991) *Computers for Social Change and Community Organizing*. New York, The Haworth Press, Inc.

New Technology in the Human Services. University of Southampton, U.K. Retrieved March 19, 2000 from the World Wide Web: http://www.soton.ac.uk/~chst/nths/subscrib.htm

New Technology in Human Services Resources. Retrieved March 19, 2000 from the World Wide Web: http://www.soton.ac.uk/~chst/direct.htm

Reck, E.T. *AFTERWORD* (no date) Retrieved March 19, 2000 from the World Wide Web: http://www.tulane.edu/~tssw/Journal/afterword.htm

Schwartz, M.D. (ed) (1984) *Using Computers in Clinical Practice: Psychotherapy and Mental Health Applications*. New York, The Haworth Press, Inc.

Social Work 211: Information Technology in Social Work (no date) (Instructors Gust Mitchell and Holly Matto) University of Maryland, Baltimore (UMBC). Retrieved from the World Wide Web March 19, 2000: http://umbc7.umbc.edu/~gmitchel/211lab.htm

Social Work Access Network (Swan) (9/97) Retrieved from the World Wide Web March 19, 2000 http://www.sc.edu/swan

Software Review Form (1997) *Computers in Human Services*, Keisha Software Review Vol 14#2 51-56. Retrieved March 19, 2000 from the World Wide Web: http://members.home.net/mcfadden/images/keishrev.html

University of South Carolina, College of Social Work. *Technology Conference for Social Work Education and Practice*. Retrieved from World Wide Web March 19, 2000: http://www.sc.edu/cosw/

World Wide Web Resources for Social Workers (3/19/00) Retrieved from the World Wide Web March 19, 2000 http://www.nyu.edu/socialwork/wwwrsw/

APPENDIX

List of schools/organizations contacted

Graduate Schools

Case Western Reserve (spoke with 1 faculty; 1 staff)
Columbia University
Florida State University
New York University
Syracuse University
University of California (Berkeley)
University of Maryland
University of Nevada (Las Vegas)
University of Nevada (Reno)
University of New Hampshire
University of South Carolina
University of Utah
University of Wisconsin (Madison)
Virginia Commonwealth University

MSW Candidate School (already has BSW program)
Ohio University

Organizations and Individuals
National Association of Social Workers (NASW)
Council on Social Work Education (CSWE)
Institute for the Advancement of Social Work Research (IASWR)
Dr. Dick Schoech–University of Texas, Arlington

The Impact of Distance Education Technology on Blending Two Cultures

Priscilla R. Smith
Nikki W. Wingerson

SUMMARY. The authors describe their experiences with distance education technology as it has impacted the development of a joint MSW program's shared culture. This phenomenon is examined from a symbolic interactionist perspective which focuses on interactions, shared perspectives, contexts, participations, and meanings. While most interaction occurs in their "smart" rooms, the authors have found one-on-one and in-person interactions to be the most productive in terms of creating shared perspectives, a vital part of culture. *[Article copies available for a fee from The Haworth Document Delivery Service: 1-800-342-9678. E-mail address: <getinfo@haworthpressinc.com> Website: <http://www.HaworthPress.com> © 2001 by The Haworth Press, Inc. All rights reserved.]*

KEYWORDS. Distance education, technology, social work, culture

Two fairly recent trends, distance education and schools collaborating to offer joint programs, are beginning to occur in social work education. The literature on distance education has largely focused on describing various technologies, strategies, and questions of effectiveness. But very little has been written about more qualitative phenome-

---

Priscilla R. Smith, PhD, and Nikki W. Wingerson, PhD, are Assistant Professors at The University of Akron, School of Social Work, Polsky Building, Suite 411, Akron, OH 44325-8001.

[Haworth co-indexing entry note]: "The Impact of Distance Education Technology on Blending Two Cultures." Smith, Priscilla R., and Nikki W. Wingerson. Co-published simultaneously in *Journal of Technology in Human Services* (The Haworth Press, Inc.) Vol. 18, No. 1/2, 2001, pp. 19-31; and: *Using Technology in Human Services Education: Going the Distance* (ed: Goutham M. Menon, and Nancy K. Brown) The Haworth Press, Inc., 2001, pp. 19-31. Single or multiple copies of this article are available for a fee from The Haworth Document Delivery Service [1-800-342-9678, 9:00 a.m. - 5:00 p.m. (EST). E-mail address: getinfo@haworthpressinc.com].

na, such as the impact of technology on classroom dynamics or program culture. Understanding an organization's culture is essential to understanding an organization's "behavior." Culture is not only created in interaction, but influences interaction. This paper examines the impact of distance education technology on the developing culture of a newly accredited Master of Social Work program. This program is a joint venture of two universities which is exclusively taught via distance education technology.

CULTURE

Culture has been defined various ways in the social science literature. From a symbolic interactionist perspective, Charon states "culture means the 'consensus' of the group, the agreements, the shared understandings, the shared language and knowledge, and the rules that are supposed to govern action" (1987, p. 165). He arrives at the following definition of culture as (1) "*a shared perspective* through which individuals in interaction define reality, and (2) *a generalized other* through which individuals in interaction control their acts" (1989, p. 167). Charon differentiates culture from social structure. While both culture and structure arise from interaction and in turn influence interaction (thus forming a dialectical relationship), social structure is the patterning of relationships (p. 172). For our purposes in this paper, we use a definition of culture consistent with Charon's, which is shared perspectives and internalized guides for behavior developed through interaction.

PROGRAM DESCRIPTION

The joint MSW program is a collaboration of Cleveland State University and The University of Akron which delivers its entire curriculum via interactive videoconferencing technology (IVT). The two large urban universities are located 35 miles apart in Northeast Ohio. This program is the only public MSW program in the area. Each university maintains autonomous schools/departments which operate separate BSW programs.

While there are other joint MSW programs which may or may not use distance education technology, the most distinctive characteristic of this joint MSW program is its exclusive program delivery via distance education technology. As with other joint programs, there are several unique program structures. In our program the Director's position and the Field Coordinator's position are rotated between the two departments/schools every four years. Thus, when the Director and Field Coordinator positions are located at Cleveland State University, the Associate Director and Associate Field Coordinator are from The University of Akron. In addition, the directorship and field coordination are administered in teams to ensure continuity of leadership. Similarly, the faculty committees and student organization also have shared governance structures. Each faculty committee has co-chairs from each university. Committee reports are presented at monthly joint faculty meetings. However, unlike joint programs which are not taught via distance education technology, our program conducts faculty meetings via our respective "smart" room technology. In addition, all committee meetings, advisory/visiting committee meetings, and student organization meetings are held via IVT.

There are additional structural elements which are unique to a joint distance education program. These have been negotiated at various academic levels and include the purchasing of phone and fax equipment for the "smart" rooms, technological support for this equipment, extensive use of e-mail and conference calling, overnight/express mail, and combined face-to-face orientation for incoming students. These negotiations required compromises, concessions, and creativity, largely from the administrators with faculty input.

The faculty and student compositions have been quite similar with regards to experience with distance education. No student had prior experience with distance education, but each student was oriented to the "smart room" prior to the start of classes. No faculty had teaching experience with either distance education or joint programs. Several distance education training sessions for faculty have been offered at different points in time, beginning with a workshop conducted by an outside expert prior to faculty delivering classes.

CONTEXTS

Since interaction gives rise to culture (shared perspectives and generalized guides for action) and structure, the contexts of those interactions need to be identified. Relevant contexts which influence the development of our blended culture and program structure can be categorized as political, professional, institutional, and physical.

Political

The political context in which our program was formed was (1) the Ohio Board of Regents required collaboration in new program development and (2) state funds for higher education were decreased. Since both Cleveland State University and The University of Akron wanted MSW programs, collaboration became necessary. This context has influenced interactions as the participants bring high levels of commitment to the table.

Professional

The professional context which influences our interactions and, therefore, development of program culture and structure is the Council on Social Work Education (CSWE). To be a viable program, we must be accredited by this body. Thus, compliance with the Council's standards and the required self-study direct much of the content of our discussions, as well as the ways we participate with each other. Therefore, all meetings (faculty, advisory, student organization, and committee) occur in the professional context of accreditation from CSWE.

Institutional

The various dual institutional contexts (two universities, two graduate schools, two colleges, and two schools/departments) also influence the interactions which give rise to culture and structure. Each of these bodies have policies. Thus, the grading system which the joint program adopted had to be created from different existing policies. This system had to be negotiated and approved at various levels of both universities, beginning at the school/department level of directors and faculty. Since culture and structure change significantly with much difficulty, faculty have been reluctant to entertain, let alone adopt, perspectives and policies different from their respective BSW programs. Similar processes occurred in developing other aspects of the program mentioned earlier.

Physical

Physically, the MSW program originates from two separate locations. The distance from the smart room to the department/school and faculty offices is much greater at one university than at the other, where all are located not only in the same building, but on the same floor. Thus, on-site faculty are more readily accessible at one university, a fact of which students at both sites are aware.

TECHNOLOGY AS CONTEXT

In a distance education program, one of the major contexts is the technology. The nature of interaction among participants involves television monitors, microphones, computer e-mail, telephones, conference calls, and overnight/express mail. The primary vehicle for teaching program content and conducting meetings of any sort is the "smart" room. Currently one such room is utilized at each site. Even this term for this room was not initially used by both faculties. The universal use of the term "smart" room took time. Gradually, a shared perspective emerged relative to the educational process taking place in that room: students learn to be "smart" professionals and we, faculty, experience mastery in the realms of technology-based teaching and masters level curriculum development. Students take every class, on their respective campuses, in the "smart" room. They sit in chairs at tables upon which microphones are placed and face the lectern, two TV monitors, and a camera. One monitor shows their off-site student colleagues, the other themselves (so they need not turn around to converse with their on-site classmates behind them). An instructor may teach from either site. Students at the site where the instructor is off site can "tune-in" the teacher via a control panel near the lectern (or ask the teacher to do so for them). The instructor teaching the class composed of on- and off-site students hears and sees the off-site students in a monitor facing the lectern. A camera on top of this monitor sends the faculty image to the other site and sound equipment sends her/his voice. Or the faculty can choose from a number of cameras via a control panel near the lectern to send: a live picture of the students s/he is with, a videotape, a Power Point presentation, a connection to the Web, or an image from the document camera. Sound accompanies all of these images.

Each "smart" room has a phone so students can call the course instructor or their off-site student colleagues during class breaks for private, individualized discussion. Students and faculty use e-mail and other telephones for the same purpose. Course materials are transported between campuses by overnight/express mail or faculty traveling to the alternate site. Sometimes even the office fax machine is utilized for this purpose. The use of technology requires all faculty to be prepared ahead of time and all students to be tolerant of delayed materials. These universal experiences have been fodder for discussions which have resulted in shared perspectives about the challenges posed by distance education technology.

Initially, differences in the equipment and technical support staff at each site impacted interaction and underscored the fact that the "smart" rooms were located at two separate universities. Use of the equipment, overall, was a cohesive force for students and for faculty, but loyalty to one's own school/department prompted the casting of comparisons about the equipment or support in terms negative towards the other site: "We invested in larger monitors than you did, and you reap the benefits of clearer visual perception" was countered by "We invested in a better audio system than you did." Gradually, as faculty taught from the alternate site and experienced the pros and cons of each set of equipment, a shared perspective emerged. This focused less on equipment differences and more on the importance of using each set of equipment to full advantage, as well as in-person, phone, and e-mail contact with alternate site students and faculty.

Differences in availability and proximity of technology support staff has impacted classroom interaction and also highlighted the fact that two universities are involved in this enterprise. When equipment fails and the off-site class loses their connection with the instructor and half the class, students and faculty alike become frustrated and negative. This is exacerbated by the fact that only one site has nearby, accessible technological help. In addition, neither site has a facilitator of any kind in the off-site classroom to help resolve equipment failures. On the positive side, faculty are confronted with difficulties daily and forced to work them out. This creates a universal experience. When faculty discuss these experiences, shared perspectives and generalized guides for action develop, and the culture building continues.

Our culture is being developed in a technological context. Use of distance education technology in teaching has been a source of anxiety, frustration, and gradually developing faculty pride. In the process of learning about the factors which make for excellence in distance education teaching, faculty have become aware of their teaching skills, generally, and ways to improve them. For example, drawing off-site students into classroom interaction requires planning relevant participatory exercises, noticing student cues of interest or disinterest, calling on students by name, and helping students draw conclusions from discussion. We are beginning to share these insights with each other, thus developing our own teaching culture as part of the program culture. However, same-site faculty have a longer shared history and culture, and are proximal to one another, inviting revelation. Thus, while faculty have experienced the technology as new at generally the same time, and many have a heightened awareness of their skills, discussion about this has essentially been with same-site faculty, perhaps contributing to the development of site subcultures.

The majority of in-person interaction is replaced by IVT communication. Frequently, the nature of interactions characteristic of distance education–largely neither in-person, nor one-on-one–is tense. In fact, the strained relations, or "site-tension" (Rooney, Izaksonas, & Macy, 1998, p. 274) noted between distance site student cohorts can be seen in polarized, stereotyped faculty perceptions and associated interactions. Under these circumstances, smooth development of a shared culture is difficult. In sum, this technological context has strongly influenced our interactions and subsequently our perspectives as part of the culture we are developing.

PERSPECTIVES

Shared perspectives are one of the two major components of culture according to Charon (1989, p. 172), as discussed earlier. These perspectives arise from interaction of the participants. The most significant participants in developing our program culture are the Program Director and Associate Director, the Field Coordinators, the students, staff, and to a lesser extent, the technicians, deans, and university presidents.

The shared perspectives of the program leaders regarding technology are extremely influential in developing program culture and need to be identified. While perspectives cannot be "seen," evidence of them can be observed. An important shared perspective of the Directors is that one aspect of the program mission–to make graduate social work education accessible in Northeast Ohio–is furthered by distance education technology. Also, the Directors share a perspective that technology should be used so as to minimize potential competition between the academic units. This is evidenced by the Associate Director's decision not to serve the members of the visiting committee lunch in one "smart" room so the members of the visiting committee at the other site (which has less funds for such expenses) would not see this over IVT.

The leaders also share the view that the program is a partnership. Related to the partnership view is a shared perspective of the need for reciprocity between the two departments/schools. The incremental upgrading of equipment by both sides has always been guided by the perspective that both sites should have as similar technologies as possible.

The program leaders recognized and agreed upon the vital importance of compromise and relinquishing school/department autonomy in this joint program endeavor. With regards to different perspectives, Charon (1989) states:

> culture is negotiated . . . Negotiation means that something among actors emerges out of the acts of all to each other. Each does not get his or her own way exactly, but instead the input by each affects the net result to some extent. Ideas, rules, direction of the group, direction of the individuals–all are negotiated in interaction. (p. 169)

The Directors also expressed the view that issues which would create barriers needed to be dealt with. Such issues included equipment and faculty traveling between sites. While most of these issues were negotiated by administrators, some have been negotiated by faculty. Discussions between the two site faculty have been conducted via IVT, while same site faculty discussions took place in person in hallways and offices. Field coordinator and committee co-chair discussions occurred on the phone and in person.

Students also have developed some shared perspectives through negotiation via technology. Not only do students of different campuses have different views, but on some issues, differences are more associated with day vs. night experiences or macro vs. micro concentrations. Unlike the faculty and staff, they are not part of two distinct programs (MSW and BSW–one distance education, one not). In some ways this enables forming shared perspectives more readily. Some of the shared perspectives the students have developed about learning in a distance education environment include the advantages of muting the sound at their respective sites during breaks. Some student co-presidents view frequent contact with each other as critical and this is evidenced by numerous calls, e-mails, and meetings.

MEANINGS

A concept related to perspectives is meanings. A synonym for meaning in this context might be significance. If something is meaningful to a person, it represents or stands for something to them (Charon, 1989, p. 40). In terms of developing a blended culture via technology, our joint MSW program means different things to the various participants. For our directors it means increased recognition of their respective school/department for delivering a joint masters program totally through distance education technology. For our university presidents, it means they can claim a university sharing the only joint totally distance education MSW program in the country. Meanings, too, are not only developed in various contexts and interactions, but are maintained and changed through interaction. Thus, as the culture continues to develop, so do meanings as a part of that culture.

PARTICIPATIONS

In addition to contexts, the ways actors participate with each other (participations) influence their interactions. In addition to classroom education, other participations include meetings (faculty, student, advisory, committee), faculty trainings, phone conversations, student orientations, faculty retreats, chance encounters, ceremonies, and social events. The first two, meetings and faculty trainings, occur exclusively in the "smart" rooms and comprise the vast majority of the participants' time together. Phone conversations and student orientations occur both in and out of the "smart" rooms. The last four all occur in-person and/or one-on-one, but these interactions are infrequent.

Meetings

Due to the unique features of this program, student and faculty teamwork and meetings are frequently organized outside of the "smart" rooms, but meetings are held in the "smart" rooms. Site tension is evidenced here by same-site faculty writing notes to each other and complaining in the halls about offensive off-site faculty behavior during meetings. Site tension during these meetings has been lessened by the even-handed stance of the program leadership. Despite the tension, evidence of shared culture has emerged from these interactions, for example in the decision-making realm. Decisions tend to be made by consensus, rather than voting as stipulated in the By Laws.

Committee meetings are usually held in the "smart" rooms, though sometimes faculty have chosen to meet in person to work together on long projects. These committees are co-chaired by representatives from, and have equal representation from, each faculty. Chairs of the committees have, of necessity, been both junior and senior faculty. Decisions about "who is to work on what" are complicated by the fact that junior faculty have had less university teaching experience. Meetings have often been very difficult in that empathy and understanding regarding the views and behaviors of off-site faculty, of any rank, has developed slowly. Decisions about meeting times are made more difficult because the "smart" room itself is available on a limited basis.

Faculty Training

Joint training experiences provide a basis for developing shared perspectives about teaching via distance education. Training in the use of distance education technology has been held with same-site faculty and with all program faculty combined. To date, faculty in a same-site training have been more apt to reveal their technological fears and tribulations.

Retreats, Encounters, and Orientations

Faculty retreats and even brief chance encounters among cross-site faculty in the halls have enabled faculty to get to know each other better as "one of us." An all-day faculty retreat at one of the two universities focused on preparation for a CSWE accreditation site visit and was anticipated with almost universal dread. However, a sense of faculty exhilaration was generated at the retreat by the shared focus, in-person interaction, and shared accomplishment. This experience highlighted for all concerned the importance of building in-person interaction into the program. This importance is further evidenced by the fact that orientation for incoming students is done on an in-person, whole class basis.

Social Events

One particular site has traditionally had a holiday party away from campus and now invites faculty from the other site, who have had no off-campus party. These other site faculty have generally opted not to attend this party, preferring less organized and smaller social encounters with their own site faculty, such as lunches or performing arts events.

Thus, the various ways we participate with each other has influenced our interactions and, in turn, our perspectives. The bulk of our participations have occurred within the "smart" rooms. Minimal participations have occurred in person or one-on-one. Yet the latter have resulted in human connections which have contributed significantly to building a shared culture.

LESSONS LEARNED

Our experiences have provided us with some practical knowledge about cultivating a shared culture. A joint distance education program needs to have the support and commitment of both universities' administrators in terms of roughly comparable technological resources (facilities and equipment). New full- and part-time faculty must have comprehensive training in the use of distance education technology. All faculty need training and ongoing distance education workshops in the use of updated technology. Conflict and struggles over variances in equipment and procedures between the two sites are inevitable and potentially beneficial. Universal struggles provide a historical basis for developing a new culture. In addition, particular shared perspectives of the program leaders about technology not only impact their interaction and negotiations, but also those of faculty and students.

While the various participants come to the program with different goals (e.g., get a degree, teach at the MSW level), all share the perspective that an MSW program is necessary to achieve these goals. Collaboration was a requirement for getting our MSW program started. That requirement alone is not sufficient motivation for the sustained interaction necessary for developing a distance education program and culture.

Meanings, which develop through interactions and shared perspectives, in turn encourage us to continue interacting. This becomes particularly significant at various times such as during the accreditation process and the immediate post-accreditation period. So, we suggest that those who are talking with each other over the monitors keep talking. Talk not only about the task at hand but also about the process. The difficulty of communicating through distance education technology makes conversation more challenging, but also more essential.

In terms of kinds of interactions, those who have developed shared perspectives faster (e.g., the Program Directors, the Field Coordinators, committee co-chairs) have had the most frequent one-on-one contact, especially face-to-face. One-on-one contact is also important for faculty and students. Face-to-face contact, such as faculty retreats, student orientations, and same-site class sessions, has been equally valuable. In-person faculty retreats, at least annually, foster greater understanding and shared perspectives.

IMPLICATIONS FOR SOCIAL WORK EDUCATION

From our experience, the technology of distance education is the characteristic which emerges as dominating the process of blending two cultures in an MSW program. As culture is comprised of shared perspectives and generalized guides for action (Charon, 1989), program culture becomes stronger and more defined as the number of shared perspectives increases about delivering and working in an MSW program, about distance education, and about shared social work programs. These perspectives become shared only through interaction. These interactions occur in various contexts (political, professional, institutional, and physical). These interactions also give rise to various meanings held by participants about the program and its developing culture. While our program is solely delivered and largely faculty governed via distance education technology, we have found some of the most productive interactions, in terms of developing shared perspectives, are one-on-one and/or in-person in nature. This is evidenced by the kinds of working relationships, policies, and procedures which follow these types of interactions. In other words, while we acknowledge the benefits of distance education such as accessibility, those interactions which do not use distance education technology are ironically the most beneficial to developing a shared culture. However, we suggest not circumventing technology, such as reducing use of the smart rooms, but augmenting the technology with one-on-one and face-to-face interactions. To facilitate the blending of cultures between social work programs which utilize distance education technology, contact between sites needs to be increased, especially in-person and one-on-one.

REFERENCES

Charon, J. M. (1989). *Symbolic interactionism: An introduction, an interpretation, an integration* (3rd ed.). Englewood Cliffs, NJ: Prentice-Hall.

Rooney, R. H., Izaksonas, E., & Macy, J. A. (1998). Reframing from site bias to site identity: Pedagogic issues in delivering social work courses via interactive television. In *Proceedings of the Conference on Information Technologies for Social Work Education*, 272-282.

Successful Distance Learning Graduate Education in Human Services

John J. Newhouse

SUMMARY. There is a critical learning process unique to graduate human services education. This process needs to be applied in the distance-learning environment. The planning and designing of course material, along with instructional strategies, need to incorporate the five phases of this learning process. Faculty who use this process to develop and deliver their distance programs will utilize the technology and educational environment of distance learning to the fullest. This paper gives readers the framework for designing human services courses so that graduate students benefit from the structure and presentation of course material in the unique environment of distance learning. *[Article copies available for a fee from The Haworth Document Delivery Service: 1-800-342-9678. E-mail address: <getinfo@haworthpressinc.com> Website: <http://www.HaworthPress.com> © 2001 by The Haworth Press, Inc. All rights reserved.]*

KEYWORDS. Distance education, distance learning, graduate education

Distance learning and graduate education are not strangers. For the past 30 years graduate level courses have been delivered through some distance learning method (Okula, 1999; Maxwell & Others, 1995). The technology of distance learning has continuously improved through the use of more sophisticated video, audio, and computer

---

John J. Newhouse, MS, MEd, EdD, is Assistant Professor, Saint Joseph's University, Department of Health Services, 5600 City Avenue, Philadelphia, PA 19131.

[Haworth co-indexing entry note]: "Successful Distance Learning Graduate Education in Human Services." Newhouse, John J. Co-published simultaneously in *Journal of Technology in Human Services* (The Haworth Press, Inc.) Vol. 18, No. 1/2, 2001, pp. 33-50; and: *Using Technology in Human Services Education: Going the Distance* (ed: Goutham M. Menon, and Nancy K. Brown) The Haworth Press, Inc., 2001, pp. 33-50. Single or multiple copies of this article are available for a fee from The Haworth Document Delivery Service [1-800-342-9678, 9:00 a.m. - 5:00 p.m. (EST). E-mail address: getinfo@haworthpressinc.com].

technology, but the principle elements of distance learning have remained constant. Simultaneous learning can occur at multiple sites regardless of the distances between these sites with one faculty member managing the course's educational process. Over time this principle has been applied to video conferencing, teleconferencing, and complete interactive video/audio transmission. One could argue that distance learning also represented the earlier technologies of one-way video and audio transmission. It is not difficult to trace the evolution of distance learning through its technological advances. What is less understood is how teaching strategies and methodologies have changed as a result of the technical advances in the field (Gee, 1990; Olcott, 1997).

For faculty in the graduate human services field the question is how to design, structure, and deliver quality education through the medium of distance learning. At the root of this assignment is the understanding that there is a critical learning process unique to graduate human services education. The uniqueness comes in two ways. First, graduate human services disciplines relate the theory of their fields to the practice in their fields. Human services education is practice based on a theoretical model (Vayda & Bogo, 1991). The educational goal is to have students integrate theory and practice so that a unifying model of professional decision-making, critical analysis, and interventional strategy application can be delivered in the work environment. The second aspect of uniqueness deals with the nature of adult learners as graduate students and what they need to experience to achieve the necessary knowledge and information. David Kolb in 1984 expressed this dynamic well with his four-stage cycle of learning. Kolb's construct began with concrete experience followed by observation and reflection. This led to the formulation of abstract concepts and hypotheses to be tested in future action. Finally, these abstract concepts and hypotheses led to new experience making the cycle complete (Kolb, 1984). The critical learning process for graduate human services education is based upon the understanding that human services fields are action oriented based upon theoretical foundations, and that graduate students are adult learners needing to reference their learning based upon their experience. They use this experience for new knowledge.

Returning to the initial question, what are the specific teaching practices and strategies that human services require when its content is being delivered through distance learning? All teaching/learning environments have limitations; all provide certain opportunities (Angelo,

1993). Distance learning removes the personal face-to-face exposure of the faculty member with students not at the site where the faculty member is present, often referred to as the far side. For graduate education in human services this limitation of distance learning could result in reduced face-to-face instructional effectiveness, lower student satisfaction, or poorer student performance (Diaz & Cartnal, 1999). This would be the case if the instructor was unskilled in distance learning technology, unaware of learning styles that are more conducive to distance learning, or simply inhibited and uneasy in its application. In any case a distance-learning course in human services would run the risk of not achieving its learning objectives (Egan & Gibb, 1997). But the very nature of distance learning that may cause issues for instructor and student interaction is the basis for valuable learning opportunities. With students at remote or far side locations there is the real possibility for richer exchanges of ideas and critical thinking that can enhance graduate human services education.

Human services made up of social work, public administration, public health, and health care has several core educational goals. Students studying these disciplines need to understand the scope of these fields and the organizational structures they contain. Other critical areas are how historical developments have impacted the field's current structure. What external pressures, whether economic, political, regulatory, legal, ethical or social, are forcing changes? Another content category represents the theoretical underpinnings of the field. Each human service discipline is based in part upon some psychosocial, social and economic theory. Students have to gain this fundamental knowledge in order to relate to the more application-based information that represents the delivery of services in these fields. Finally, each human services discipline has numerous practice systems and functional areas. The professional development of graduate students requires them to have a working knowledge of the business or operational areas needed to deliver services. These three major content pieces–scope, theory, and practice–are what faculty address in the courses they teach.

COURSE CONTENT AND INSTRUCTIONAL APPROACHES

Planning and designing graduate human services curriculum in a distance-learning environment begins with the awareness that course content will represent some combination of scope, theory, and practice. The mix of these three content areas varies, but it's important in the instructional design function to recognize where and when each area occurs. This understanding is critical for the faculty member as he/she plans how to design a distance learning course program. Regardless of the level of technology a distance-learning environment represents, there are several instructional strategies available to the instructor. The faculty member can present content information to the entire class population as a large group audience. Students can engage in an open dialogue as an entire class exchanging opinions and providing each other with feedback (McHenry & Bozik, 1995). Students can work in small groups or teams requiring critical analysis and the completion of specific assignments. Individual students can be asked to present the results of their work to the whole class. Students can be asked to role-play case situations in a variety of formats–individual, small groups, dyads (Nilson, 1998). The result is that faculty have these key approaches to consider in their distance learning planning process: presentations, discussions, group work, and role plays (see Figure 1). It now becomes a question of how to apply distance-learning technology in its environment to best achieve learning outcomes for any of these approaches.

FIVE INSTRUCTIONAL PROCESS PHASES

There are five instructional process phases or steps that graduate students experience as they gain the scope, theory, and practice of their human services field. Students acquire and process the information they are given (Clark & Robinson, 1994; Saba & Shearer, 1994). They will automatically move through these phases whether or not the faculty member has consciously designed the instructional process with these steps in mind. This happens because of the very nature of adult education and is outside the control of the instructor (Wagschal & Wagschal, 1995). Using this reality to develop a distance learning program model results in courses that students feel are well structured and provides them with new knowledge they previously did not have. This model reflects the major tenets of the cognitive theories based on constructivism and transformative learning. In constructivism theory learning happens through information processing and the process of knowledge-construction requires learners to be active in developing

FIGURE 1. Instructional Approaches for Distance Learning

Instructional Approaches		Applications
1.	Presentations	Instructor presentation to entire class Individual student presentation to entire class Small group presentation to entire class
2.	Discussions	Large group, open discussion for entire class Open group discussion at each location
3.	Group Work	Group assignment to complete an exercise Group assignment to conduct a simulation Group assignment to discuss a topic, content, article, text material, handout Group assignment to develop a presentation
4.	Role Plays	Role play for two students Role play for three to five students Role play with one or more students serving as observers

their own understanding of the topics they study. Constructivism, as a learning theory, has five characteristics: (1) only those engaged in the learning can construct their own understanding of that which is being learned; (2) new knowledge depends on prior understanding of the information and content; (3) all learning results from conceptual change in the mind of the learner; (4) understanding is achieved within a social context; and (5) meaningful learning occurs within authentic learning tasks (Eggen, 1995). For this five-phase distance learning approach to succeed there must be new opportunities for interactivity to occur. Costas Spirou, a colleague of Paul Eggen in the field of college teaching and learning, notes the importance of interactivity to achieve meaningful learning and positive student experiences. Spirou writes:

> The development of an appropriate distance teaching pedagogy could produce, in addition to teacher-student interaction, an opportunity for student-student interaction across multiple sites. This in turn would generate an environment in which technology itself becomes secondary to the exchange of ideas. (Spirou, 1995, p. 134)

Supplementing constructivism in this five-step distance-learning model is transformative learning theory. This theory views learning as a process of becoming aware of one's assumptions and revising these assumptions based on critical self-reflection. This self-reflection allows the students to question assumptions, decide the degree of validity these assumptions have, and then develop new ways of interpreting the world around them. Their changed perspectives ultimately change their actions and their behaviors (Cranton, 1994). Constructivism provides the interactivity so critical for this model, while transformative learning theory provides the necessary reflection that runs from phase two through all other phases to the final one. In this distance learning model students confront existing assumptions about the content being taught. For adults such confrontation is essential. Cranton writes, "If basic assumptions are not challenged, change will not take place" (Cranton, 1994, p. 739). Such critical self-reflection is achieved through the instructional design and implementation of this distance-learning model. The elements of constructivism and transformative learning that combine to form the foundation of this five phase distance learning model also argue for effective learning and knowledge retention. Ference Marton in his studies in 1979 and 1983 consistently found that college students who defined the content of their academic subjects in terms of their surrounding world experienced this knowledge as part of themselves or as a change in the way they conceptualized their environment. Students who approached learning in this way achieved greater depth of knowledge and increased retention (Marton, 1979; Marton, 1983). Similar results were obtained through the work of Wingfield (1979) and later confirmed by Houston (1981). Wingfield showed that through levels of cognitive processing material continually undergoes varying degrees of analysis as it is being related to knowledge already in the memory. This supports the premise of constructivism as a learning process engaged with interactivity between what is being learned and what has already been learned. It also supports transformative learning theory with its commitment to self-reflection as the means for transforming one's learned outcomes.

Content presentation is the first of the five process phases in the graduate education distance-learning model for human services. Normally, this is done through an instructor's presentation to the entire class. Common human services content presented in this phase is the field's historical components, the field's scope, and its theoretical basis. Faculty members present those pieces of this content they deem necessary for the course program. Additional information may be presented by individual students or students working in small groups.

The key for this first process phase is that information is being communicated to students in mostly a one-way direction for their comprehension.

Step two involves the students' processing of this information. Processing means the ability of the students to listen and understand what is being presented. They need to gain a clear mental concept of this information. They need to feel comfortable with their level of clarity and understanding. Phase two is about confirming the meaning of this information in its uncensored form. It's what Wingfield would call levels of processing (Wingfield, 1979). Faculty members or student presenters can expect questions and the need to clarify their content during this phase. Once this has been done and students have a firm understanding of the content, they are ready to move to the third step. It is at this third process phase that the graduate students' professional work experience is first involved.

In step three students are comparing what they have just learned with their own understanding of work and professional life. It is a form of validation in which the presented information is being assessed against what has been experienced or observed in the work setting. As stated above, the principles of constructivism are occurring. It is difficult for faculty to see this process happening, but student comments and body language are ways to know that students are working through this third phase. It is critical in the instructional process journey since it confirms in the student's mind that this information has relevance to his/her career in this particular human services field.

Once validation has occurred, students move to exploring how this newly acquired information and knowledge can be applied. In this fourth step the critical student behavior is the analysis of options. Students want to understand how this information can be tailored to their situations. Transformative learning takes over in this fourth phase. It may be that students will find no immediate use for this new knowledge. It could be a limited application that they discover. What is critical is that the information not be lost or forgotten if it is seen as usable. Graduate students perceive a high value between what they learn in formal education and what they can use (Still & Kent, 1995). This step is about that relationship.

The final process step occurs when a student decides to imagine how a particular application of the information would actually work. It is analogous to market testing for a new service or product. In this case testing of the application or utilization is being done through mental imaging as a mock approach. Again, transformative learning theory is at the core of this phase. The student has surveyed the possibilities through his/her exploration in phase four and now the attempt is being made to mentally apply all of the information or portions of it to determine its effectiveness. This is the application process that will move the course material from the classroom to the work environment. It could happen the next day after class or it might happen several days or weeks later. The critical issue is that some aspect of the new information and knowledge presented in process step one, is now ready for application in the student's professional life. This is the ultimate reason for human services graduate education. It's the point at which the student feels most fulfilled from the course's content.

PROCESS PHASE CHALLENGES

From the instructor's perspective, these five instructional process phases have specific challenges. In the distance-learning environment it would seem as if the entire technology has been developed to enhance content presentation. Even in the relatively basic distance learning settings there is interactive video and audio capability (Thach & Murphy, 1995). Material can be presented live. It can be done using computer programs; it can be done using all types of media. The challenge for the faculty member is *choosing what to use* that will produce the best comprehension and retention rate for the students. Phase two has the challenge that *each student represents different levels of experience* in terms of the information being presented. It can be seen as a continuum from little or no experience at one end to considerable experience at the other. Distance learning can enhance the student's ability to understand and comprehend what is being presented since there are more opportunities to exchange ideas and opinions with multiple class populations. The challenge in the validation phase is to allow students the *time to make this assessment*. It can be almost instantaneous for some students and prolonged for others. As students recall their work experience and survey what they have seen and done, they may need to cover this ground carefully and deliberately. Using examples or mini-cases may help students make their own connections. It's important that faculty allow this to happen. In phase four faculty face the challenge of *creating an open-ended learning environment.* As students explore what are potential uses and application of this new knowledge and information for their professional lives, they need to experience an educational setting that is non-judgmental, and welcomes this type of exploration. The faculty member has a major role to play in creating this type of environment. The final phase is the mock application of the approach the student decides to take. The challenge in this final step is *to provide the student with sufficient space to create that mental model* and determine how it would work. Phase five is the culmination of both content presentation and student response to all that has gone before. Giving students the opportunity for decision-making about the course content, brings them full circle in their new knowledge. Graduate human services education takes these five instructional process phases, their accompanying challenges, and matches process phases with distance learning instructional approaches. This construct is the design model faculty can use to develop their course programs (see Figure 2).

CONTENT AND INSTRUCTIONAL DESIGN SCOPE

The instructional design for all five phases requires that the faculty member plan the pace and the presentation of material. Since students can move through the five phases at different rates, the material needs to be structured and delivered to allow for these phases to happen. There are differences in the degree to which this is needed based upon the kind of information being taught. In most cases, when the content deals with scope within a human services field, there is less time required for students to move from the content presentation phase through the mock application phase. It also means that the organization of the content can be in larger units with fewer divisions. More can be presented, processed, validated, explored, and mentally applied than with either theory or practice types of content. It is didactic and telling a story of what is, how it came to be that way, and what components it represents. Scope information requires less analysis on the student's part. It often involves historical, social, ethical, political, regulatory, legal, and economic components. Students take this knowledge more for its contextual and foundational value than for its application. Therefore, faculty members can design those portions of the program with broader sections and fewer stopping points. This material should use the dramatic power of distance learning's technology to

FIGURE 2. Design Model for Human Services Graduate Education–Distance Learning

Phases	Challenges	Distance Learning Instructional Approaches
1. Content Presentation	Comprehension and retention rate	Instructor presents to entire class Individual student presents to entire class Small group presentation to entire class
2. Information Processing	Different student levels of experience	Open, large group discussion for entire class Open group discussion at each distance learning location Group assignment to discuss topic or content
3. Validation	Time to make an assessment	Large group, open discussion for entire class Open group discussion at each distance learning location Group assignment to discuss topic or content
4. Exploration	Creating an open ended learning environment	Open group discussion at each distance learning location Group assignment to discuss topic or content Group assignment to develop presentation to entire class Group assignment to complete exercise
5. Mock Application	Provide space to create a mental model	Group assignment to complete exercise Group assignment to conduct simulation Group assignment to discuss topic or content Role play for two students Role play for three to five students Role play with one or more students serving as observers

create impact. Sufficient planning needs to be done so that this type of information gains students' attention, and keeps them alert and able to retain what is being presented. This instructional design recommendation also applies in the case of individual students presenting scope information, such as a case review. It certainly applies when small teams of students are presenting as a group. Often students who are presenting have little sensitivity about what kind of information they are bringing to the course program. They often do not distinguish between the categories of scope, theory, or practice as different types of content material. But faculties do need to know this difference and appreciate the importance of this distinction when planning, developing, and delivering distance-learning curriculum. Here are suggestions for designing scope information that works well in the distance-learning environment.

First–Group content into major categories as one presentation
Second–Highlight the important concepts and information within the body of the presentation
Third–Conclude the presentation with summary points or learning take-aways

THEORY

Theory type content moves students through the five educational phases in continuous fashion dealing with more abstract information. Students hear and see what the theory represents and they then begin to process this information. Their processing requires that all of the remaining steps be followed. First, it is a question of validation. Can they see how this theory has been in place in their professional lives? Can they understand how this theory has helped shape their work environment and determined certain courses of action? Quickly following the validation phase is the exploration phase. Now students are questioning how this theory has been applied, for what purpose, and if a different application were done, what results would occur. This exploration of theory is the 'what if' point. Students need time to do this with theoretical information. This allows them time to understand at a conceptual level what they may have known on an experiential plane. It gives them the necessary skills to move to phase five–mock application. For theoretical information, the mock application phase takes the subjunctive thinking of phase four and turns it into working blueprints. Theory is understood and validated. It has been explored in terms of application and use. Now it has become a plan for on-going human services practice. What was unrecognized or unknown in the work environment has now become a method to forecast and plan the future. Theory content of course programs requires all five phases for the students' maximum learning. In the distance learning environment these recommendations will help design effective instruction for theoretical information.

First–Present the theory as a whole initially, informing students that it will be broken down into appropriate sub-units
Second–Deliver the theory's sub-units in a logical, cumulative fashion
Third–Allow students to move through phases 2-5 after each sub-unit has been presented
Fourth–Complete the theoretical component by connecting all of the theory's sub-units into its original form

Any of the recommended distance learning instructional approaches can be used for this type of information. The two-group discussion approaches in Figure 2 work well for theoretical information.

PRACTICE

Practice is the last type of human services course content. This, like the theory information, relies heavily on students being able to move through all five learning phases. Practice or the ability to transfer what is learned in the formal setting to the work site is crucial in adult education. Graduate students receive the information from faculty and other student presentations. Immediately, they begin their processing of this information based upon their own level of experience with it. This first post-presentation phase runs through a catalog of what they have seen and experienced with what is being suggested as practice. Matches and mismatches are being noted and remembered. Faculty needs to make the necessary time to allow students this processing opportunity. Students commit to understand exactly what is being presented. They move directly into the validation phase, asking themselves will this work and how. All points of practice both large and small are being processed. Some students discard portions of the practice information. Some choose to discard it all. In most cases students will determine for themselves its level of validation and move on to exploration.

Again, graduate students are doing serious work in this phase. They are deciding to what extent they will accept this practice information and what it means to do so. It could be described as a mental commitment based upon individual selection criteria. Phase four works through this exploration, accepting, rejecting, piecing together, and rearranging what had been validated earlier. As this process continues, students begin to enter the final learning phase. They begin to mentally apply their practice model to their own professional situations. It is the culmination of this process that results in behavioral change and successful human services graduate education. In the distance learning environment designing for practice information means that faculty build time into the process allowing this to happen. These guidelines may help in the design of practice information for distance learning programs.

First–Provide space or time after each piece of the practice has been presented
Second–Provide space or time at the end of the practice information section
Third–Use a variety of the distance learning instructional approaches for the time breaks between practice information

The following case provides an example of how this five-phase distance-learning model might be used for human services graduate education. This particular course deals with managed care, one of this country's leading health care topics and trends. A major educational goal for the course is to have students understand the key principles of managed care practice. One example of this practice theory is that managed care functions through contracted network care providers. Individual managed care organizations sign contracts for health care services at discounted prices for their subscribers. Subscribers need to use these network facilities to avoid out-of-pocket charges not covered by their managed care organization.

Phase one–Content Presentation
Challenge–Gain comprehension and increase retention rate
Distance Learning Instructional Approach–Instructor leads presentation, small group presentations

Instructor uses graphically designed material on a computer program to illustrate all components of what managed care theory represents. Instructor informs class that each component will be addressed separately. To assess learning and retention, the instructor asks students to divide into small teams at their site locations. Instructor assigns each team one aspect of managed care practice theory, giving them the assignment to discuss what the theoretical component means in practical terms for patients, care providers, and the managed care organizations. Each team is then asked to give a five minute presentation on the results of their discussions.

Phase two–Information Processing
Challenge–Accommodating different student levels of experience
Distance Learning Instructional Approach–Large group, open discussion for entire class

Instructor singles out one of the practice theory components that had been presented by one small team. The entire class (all distance learning locations) are asked to openly discuss what this component means in the world of patients, doctors, hospitals, other care givers, and third party payers. Students are encouraged to ask clarifying questions and to be clear on what this practice theory component means and how it works.

Phase three–Validation
Challenge–Time to make an assessment
Distance Learning Instructional Approach–Large group, open discussion for entire class

Instructor asks the entire class to think about what they already know or have experienced about this particular theoretical component. Students are encouraged to reflect on their personal knowledge, share experiences with the entire class, and determine to what degree they think this concept is valid. The richer student mix made possible by distance learning enhances this third phase of the model.

Phase four–Exploration
Challenge–Creating an open ended learning environment
Distance Learning Instructional Approach–Group assignment to complete an exercise

Instructor has the class reconfigure itself into the original small teams at each distance-learning site. All of the teams are given two questions to address. First, how do you know that this particular component is unique to managed care? Second, what aspects of this component may be found outside of managed care but within the health care field? The teams are given twenty minutes to discuss and answer these two questions. This type of exercise creates an open ended learning environment necessary for exploration.

Phase five–Mock Application
Challenge–Provide space to create a mental model
Distance Learning Instructional Approach–Role play for two students, group assignment to complete exercise

Instructor asks students to divide into groups of three with one person willing to play the role of a patient, another student to play the role of the in-take admissions counselor, and the third student to observe and take notes on what exchange will take place between the first two. The instructor gives each role group some parameters concerning their role to establish a context for the role-play. The observer students are told to capture important and telling comments, apparent attitudes, and body language. They are also given the time frame for the role-play. At the conclusion of the role-play, each observer student is asked to report on what he/she saw and heard. The thoughts of the two role-play students as they went through the exercise are also shared. As students report on observations, as well as on actual feelings they experienced during the role-play exercise, the mock application of this managed care component becomes real. Students have created a mental image of this managed care issue and it can easily be transferred to their work location. Older assumptions have been challenged or reinforced. Transformative learning has occurred, and the ability to apply what has been learned to the work environment has occurred.

Instructional design strategies for graduate education in distance learning do not differ from strategies in a self-contained class environment. What is different is that distance learning's multiple sites, greater diversity of students, high-end audio, and visual technology offer the possibility for more learning impact. Faculty members have the potential to capitalize on instructional elements only found in the distance-learning environment. Using these elements enhances graduate student learning. It is the deliberate planning and design of distance learning instruction that will result in this enhanced education (Cyrs, 1997). Distance learning will always represent this opportunity. It is up to individual faculty members to take advantage of this unique instructional environment and to create a rich, value-driven graduate human services curriculum.

REFERENCES

Abernathy, D. (1997, December). Start-up Guide to Distance Learning. *Training and Development*, pp. 39-41.

Abernathy, D. (1998, September). The WWW of Distance Learning: Who Does What and Where? *Training and Development*, pp. 29-30.

Angelo, T. (1993). Fourteen General Research Based Principles for Improving Higher Education. *American Academy of Higher Education Bulletin. 45*, 5-7.

Au, M., & Chong, C. (1993). The Evaluation of the Effectiveness of Various Distance Learning Methods. *International Journal of Instructional Media, 20* (2), 105-112.

Bagnall, G. (1995). Postgraduate Training in Health Education/Promotion: The Demand from Potential Students for Distance Learning. *The Health Education Journal. 54* (2), 63-168.

Clark, E., & Robinson, K. (1994, August). Open Learning: The State of the Art in Nursing and Midwifery. *Nurse Educator Today*, pp. 257-263.

Cranton, P. (1994, November/December). Self-Directed and Transformative Instructional Development. *Journal of Higher Education. 65* (6), 726-744.

Cyrs, T. E. (1997). Competence in Teaching at a Distance. (Monograph). *New Directions for Teaching and Learning, 71*, 15-18.

Diaz, D. P. & Cartnal, R. B. (1999). Students' Learning Styles in Two Classes. *College Teaching, 47* (4), 130-136.

Edward, N., Hugo, K., Gragg, B., & Peterson, J. (1999). The Integration of Problem-Based Learning Strategies in Distance Education. *Nurse Educator, 24* (1), 36-41.

Egan, M. W., & Gibb, G. S. (1997). Student-Centered Instruction for the Design of Telecourses. (Monograph). *New Directions for Teaching and Learning, 71*, 33-39.

Eggen, P. (1995). Learning and Motivational Theory Applied to Instruction. *Selected Papers from the Sixth National Conference on College Teaching and Learning*. (pp.59-64). Jacksonville, FL: Florida Community College.

Evans, T., & Nation, D. (1996). Theories of Teaching and Learning in Open and Distance Education. *Open Learning, 11*, (3), 50-57.

Farber, J. (1998). The Third Circle: On Education and Distance Learning. *Sociological Perspectives, 41*, (4), 797-813.

Gant, L. P. (1996). Lessons in Developing Distance Learning. *Performance + Instruction, 35*, (2), 22-26.

Gee, D. B. (1990). *The Impact of Students' Preferred Learning Style Variables in a Distance Education Course: A Case Study.* (Reports-Research/Technical-143) Lubbock, TX: Texas Tech University. (ERIC Document Reproduction Service No. ED 358836).

Gibson, C., & Gibson, T. (1995, September). Lessons Learned from 100 + Years of Distance Learning. *Adults Learning*, 15-18.

Hezel, R. T., & Nanjiani, N. (1997). Best Practices in Higher Education. *Teleconferencing Business*, *7* (5), 10, 12, 17.

Houston, J. (1981). *Fundamentals of Learning and Memory.* New York, NY: Academic Press.

Klinger, T. H., & Connet, M. R. (1992). Designing Distance Learning Courses for Critical Thinking. *The Journal-Technological Horizons in Education*, *20* (3), 87-90.

Kolb, D. (1984). *Experiential Learning: Experience as the Source of Learning and Development.* Englewood Cliffs, NJ: Prentice-Hall.

Krauth, B. (1996). Principles of Good Practice for Distance Learning Programs. *Cause/Effect*, *19* (1), 6-13.

Lohmann, J. S. (1998, September). Classrooms Without Walls: Three Companies That Took the Plunge. *Training and Development*, pp. 39-41.

Marton, F. (1979, September/October). Skill as an Aspect of Knowledge. *Journal of Higher Education*. *50* (5), 602-614.

Marton, F. (1983, May/June). Review of Student Learning in Higher Education. *Journal of Higher Education*. *54* (3), 325-329.

Maxwell, L. & Others. (1995, May). Graduate Distance Education: A Review and Synthesis of the Research Literature. *Proceedings for the Annual Conference of the International Communication Association–Instructional and Developmental Communication Division.* Albuquerque, NM.

McHenry, L., & Bozik, M. (1995). Communicating at a Distance: A Study of Interaction in a Distance Education Classroom. *Communication Education*, *44*, 362-370.

Mitkovsky, E. (1997). Techniques for Distance Learning Instruction. *Media and Methods*, *34* (1), 24.

Morgan, C. J., Dingsdaq, D., & Saenger, H. (1998). Learning Strategies for Distance Learners–Do They Help? *Distance Education*, *19* (1), 142-145.

Nilson, L. (1998). *Teaching at Its Best: A Research-Based Resource for College Instructors.* Bolton, MA: Anker Publishing Co., Inc.

Okula, S. (1999). Going the Distance–A New Avenue for Learning. *Business Education Forum*, *53* (3), 7-10.

Olcott, D., Jr. (1997). Renewing the Vision: Past Perspectives and Future Imperatives for Distance Education. *Journal of Continuing Higher Education*, *45* (3), 2-13.

Saba, F., & Shearer, R. L. (1994). Verifying Key Theoretical Concepts in a Dynamic Model of Distance Learning. *American Journal of Distance Education*, *8* (1), 36-42.

Smith, C. (1996, May). Taking the Distance Out of Distance Learning. *Training and Development*, pp. 87-89.

Spirou, C. S. (1995). Generating a Positive Student Experience in Distance Learning Education. *Selected Papers from the Sixth National Conference on College Teaching and Learning* (pp. 133-139). Jacksonville, FL: Florida Community College.

Still, G. & Kent, E. (1995). Connecting Learning and Activism: An Experiment in Adult Higher Education. *Celebrating Excellence: Learning and Teaching in Adult Higher Education–National Conference on Alternative and External Degree Programs for Adults* (pp. 131-136). Columbus, OH.

Thach, E. C., & Murphy, K. L. (1995, December). Training via Distance Learning. *Training and Development*, pp. 44-46.

Tucker, G. (1998). A Dynamic Distance Learning Program. *Media and Methods, 34* (3), 11-13.

Vayda, E. & Bogo, M. (1991). A Teaching Model to Unite Classroom and Field. *Journal of Social Work Education*, 27 (3), 271-278.

Wagschal, K. & Wagschal, P. (1995). Teaching Adult Learners. In P. Seldin (Ed.), *Improving College Teaching* (pp. 235-248). Bolton, MA: Anker Publishing Co., Inc.

Ward, E. C., & Lee, E. (1995, November). An Instructor's Guide to Distance Learning. *Training and Development*, pp. 40-44.

Webster, J., & Hackley, P. (1997). Teaching Effectiveness in Technology-Mediated Distance Learning. *Academy of Management Journal, 40* (6), 1282-1309.

Wingfield, A. (1979). *Human Learning and Memory*. New York, NY: Harper & Row.

Using Technological Tools to Enhance Learning in Social Work Diversity Courses

Marie Huff
Sherry Edwards

SUMMARY. This study explores the educational benefits of using e-mail and electronic discussion groups as instructional tools in social work diversity classes. The authors look at practical ideas of how these technological tools can be used to aid classroom instruction, increase student awareness of human diversity issues, and enhance cultural competence. Students rated their experience as positive overall, and believe it gave them more opportunity to process the course content and expand their discussions outside the classroom. Students also report that they took more time to think about their responses than they do in traditional classroom discussions. *[Article copies available for a fee from The Haworth Document Delivery Service: 1-800-342-9678. E-mail address: <getinfo@haworthpressinc.com> Website: <http://www.HaworthPress.com> © 2001 by The Haworth Press, Inc. All rights reserved.]*

KEYWORDS. Diversity, electronic mail, listserv, social work education, cultural competence

With changing world demographics, notably in the United States, social work practitioners are working more with clients who are "different" from themselves (Edwards, 1997). This demographic shift is one of the reasons that human diversity content is essential in social work

---

Marie Huff is affiliated with Western Carolina University.
Sherry Edwards is affiliated with the University of North Carolina at Pembroke.

[Haworth co-indexing entry note]: "Using Technological Tools to Enhance Learning in Social Work Diversity Courses." Huff, Marie, and Sherry Edwards. Co-published simultaneously in *Journal of Technology in Human Services* (The Haworth Press, Inc.) Vol. 18, No. 1/2, 2001, pp. 51-64; and: *Using Technology in Human Services Education: Going the Distance* (ed: Goutham M. Menon, and Nancy K. Brown) The Haworth Press, Inc., 2001, pp. 51-64. Single or multiple copies of this article are available for a fee from The Haworth Document Delivery Service [1-800-342-9678, 9:00 a.m. - 5:00 p.m. (EST). E-mail address: getinfo@haworthpressinc.com].

educational classes. Also, the Council on Social Work Education has mandated that students must be exposed to information concerning awareness about, and appreciation for, human diversity (CSWE, 1994). Accredited programs are also required to provide students with information and practice experience encompassing groups that are particularly relevant to the program's mission.

One way for educators to help students obtain this practice experience and knowledge is to use e-mail and electronic discussion groups as teaching tools. The use of electronic discussion groups and e-mail is being increasingly employed in higher education (Guernsey, 1997). Guernsey reports that out of the 605 institutions surveyed by the Campus Computing Project, one-third of the colleges utilize e-mail in their courses. The noted benefits to using electronic discussion groups as part of the class curriculum include increasing and enhancing student-student interactions, fostering a greater sense of community, and encouraging students to think about how to express their ideas in writing rather than just speaking up impulsively in class (Karayan & Crowe, 1997). Also, the electronic medium allows students to offer their opinions in a non-threatening atmosphere when they are ready to give the subject their full attention.

Edwards (1997) found that MSW students who used e-mail to submit their journal entries in a social work diversity class seemed to incorporate more of the class issues into their journals than did students who handwrote their entries. She also found that students who used e-mail wrote more often than required, and carried on more of a "dialogue" with the instructor as they processed the information and/or their own experiences. In a different study by Huff (1998), 67 percent of MSW students in a distance education class agreed that having individual e-mail journal partners enhanced their learning in their policy class.

TECHNOLOGY USED IN THE SOCIAL WORK DIVERSITY COURSES

The two human diversity courses used in this study were designed to provide the student with a theoretical perspective on human relations. The goal of each class was to aid the student to acquire a better understanding of diversity as it applies to historically oppressed and disadvantaged groups. Some of the learning objectives were to heighten students' awareness of how people get labeled in society, and the impact labeling has on the individual and society. Also, the instructors sought to enhance students' cultural awareness of how racial, ethnic, gender, sexual orientation and religious background can influence personal and professional identity, attitudes and behavior.

This cultural awareness is best presented to students when the courses offer a knowledge component, an affective component, and a practice skills component (Edwards, 1997). The use of e-mail and electronic discussion groups is one way to offer students the opportunity to become involved in affective learning, which is more likely to encourage a change in feelings, emotions, and attitudes (Meredith, Mullins, & Fortner, 1995).

Students were also given the opportunity to enhance their critical thinking skills by taking on more responsibility for their own learning and actively participating in the learning process. Paul (1990) states that students often learn best by teaching or explaining to others what they know, and by answering others' questions. The electronic discussion group and e-mail assignments were designed to increase the opportunities for students to "teach" each other by explaining what they understood from the class lectures and readings, and by asking their peers questions.

Electronic Discussion Groups

In order to expand the perspective of the students, an electronic listserv was set up between the two diversity classes. Students were instructed to post at least 10 messages on the listserv during the semester and to "initiate" at least one discussion item related to diversity issues. Because both classes were using the same text, they were able to "discuss" the same readings electronically.

The advantages of these types of communications certainly outweigh the disadvantages. Some of these advantages include: developing academic discourse, participating in collaborative and project work, maximizing the knowledge and experience of all participants, increasing equity of participation, cross-cultural participation, development of reflective writing skills, overcoming social isolation, emotional involvement, ready access to help and support, direct student contact and interactive participation, freedom from the constraints of time and location, and learner control (Edwards, 1997). Students also have the opportunity to exchange information or questions about assignments and collaborate on group projects

Electronic discussion groups allow students who are generally quiet during in-class discussions the opportunity to reflect on the readings and discussions, and then share their ideas with the class through this possibly less threatening medium (Hall, 1993). It has also been suggested that by interacting with others through the written word (e-mail and discussion groups), students are able to rise above the usually stereotypical responses to face-to-face interactions, and are able to discuss more difficult cultural issues (Jackson, Yorker, & Mitchem, 1996). Latting (1994) found an example of this in a study in which one of the students wrote, "for me, the whole medium is new. We send letters into a void, and get answers back. We're dealing with people we've never met, and have to learn without labels, which is a great experience for social worker wannabes" (p. 37). It also allows for some risk-taking comments that may not have been shared in an open classroom discussion.

Discussion and e-mail messages require students to listen and respond to the ideas of other students, something that many students do not do in the traditional classroom. Also, the writing is more informal, and many students are less intimidated as there is more emphasis on the content from their stream of consciousness. The use of technology with e-mail and discussion groups also accommodates different learning styles. It appears that students who are textual and visual do well using the on-line exchange of information (Jackson, Yorker, & Mitchem, 1996). Students are also given the opportunity to respond as they choose and are not "forced" to make immediate comments as sometimes happens in the traditional classroom.

Keyboard Pals

In addition to the listserv, all students were assigned a "keyboard pal" from the other class midway through the semester. They were to communicate with their partners weekly via individual e-mail on issues related to diversity. E-mail technology has been available for some time and is one of the most widely used computer technology applications in higher education (Lewis, Treves, & Shaindlin, 1997). E-mail applications are some of the easiest computer applications to become acquainted with. This technology has also been seen as the best and simplest place to start navigating the information highway (Banks & Coombs, 1999). As mentioned previously, students who become comfortable with this technology are more encouraged to communicate their questions and concerns to the instructor, as well as their e-mail partner, thereby enhancing their learning experience.

Students also have the availability of their "own" partner to discuss the readings assigned in class. This experience might also help to increase the students' critical thinking abilities by giving them additional opportunities to share what they know, and respond to opinions that may differ from their own. Students can also get feedback from their partner in a non-threatening environment. In addition, students have the ability to discuss assignments and other questions related to the course in order to get clarification.

This technology is especially beneficial for students who are commuting long distance to the traditional classroom and don't have easy access to their peers or faculty, as well for students who have disabilities that hinder their mobility. Banks and Coombs (1995) state, "The computer with special adaptive hardware and software is the most empowering and liberating technology to come along in decades for persons with disabilities" (p. 5). It permits students with disabilities to interact with other students and the instructor without the use of interpreters, allowing students and faculty with disabilities greater participation in the learning experience.

Several important issues were explored when considering the use of e-mail as a learning tool. First, there is the issue of confidentiality. E-mail conversations, and to some degree the listserv communications, should be treated as a private conversation unless permission is obtained from the writer to share it with others. The instructors carefully explained the risks associated with using an electronic medium, and cautioned students to think about how their messages might be interpreted before sending them out. A second issue of concern was students' comfort with the technology. Many of the students did not have personal e-mail accounts and/or did not have a home computer. Both campuses provided student access through computer labs, however, allowing students to meet the requirements of the course. The instructors also spent time with individual students who needed extra "technology tutoring."

In addition to the listserv and e-mail, there were several other occasions where students could use computer technology, but were not specifically elaborated in this study. These included such things as providing an on-line syllabus, giving web-based assignments, and electronic submission and critique of work. These learning activities also helped to make students more comfortable with the technology.

METHOD

The sample included 53 undergraduate students from two public southern universities. The majority of students were social work majors. Seventy-nine percent of them were female. Forty-eight students filled out questionnaires, 80% from one university and 100% from the other university. Although there were some differences between the two classes, instructors used the same text and similar exercises. One class met for 50 minutes 3 times a week, while the other class met once a week for three hours.

At the end of the semester, students were asked to fill out an instrument developed by the authors to measure students' perceptions regarding the effectiveness of using this type of technology in a diversity course. The students were also asked to give narrative comments regarding the learning process. There was no identifying information on the questionnaire so confidentiality was maintained. The students' listserv comments were also evaluated for themes, and for suggested improvements.

The electronic discussion group was set up at the beginning of the semester, giving students the whole semester to participate. They were not assigned their keyboard pals until the middle of the semester, after they had become relatively comfortable with using e-mail. This may have prejudiced their responses when they were asked to compare the electronic discussion group with keyboard pals.

Research Questions

The authors were interested in how using technology as a teaching tool might enhance student learning in a social work diversity class. Based on the educational literature, one would expect students to be more open expressing their opinions electronically than they might be in class during face-to-face discussions. Because exploring one's own biases and perceptions is so important when teaching diversity content, the instructors wanted to offer students a "safe" way to do this. Specifically the following research questions were addressed:

1. Do students feel more comfortable expressing their opinions electronically as opposed to open classroom discussion?
2. Does computer mediated communications enhance opportunities for learning content in social work diversity classes?
3. Does the use of computer mediated communications improve students' technology skills?
4. Does the use of computer mediated communications empower students by giving them more responsibility for their own learning?

RESULTS

The survey was divided into two sections, with students answering questions related to the electronic discussion group and the keyboard pals separately. To address the first research question, students were asked to rate their comfort level related to sharing their opinions in electronic discussion groups, keyboard pals, and in the classroom. Students were also asked to compare the listserv, keyboard pals, and the classroom forum regarding their usefulness and their own comfort level. While the majority of students felt the face-to-face discussions were the most useful for them, they reportedly felt most comfortable sharing their opinions via the listserv (Table 1).

In addition, 85% of the students agreed or strongly agreed that electronic discussion groups gave quieter students more opportunities to speak, and 83% reported being able to broach subjects that they might not bring up in class. Eighty-one percent of the students agreed

TABLE 1. Comparison of Technology Usefulness and Comfort Level–Frequency (Percentages) N = 48

Technology	Most Useful	Easiest	Comfort Sharing Opinions
Electronic Group	13 (27.1)	17 (35.4)	29 (60.4)
Keyboard Pals	1 (2.1)	21 (43.8)	7 (14.6)
Classroom	34 (70.8)	7 (14.6)	9 (18.8)
Neither		3 (6.3)	3 (6.3)

or strongly agreed that they took more time to think about their responses than they would have in a traditional classroom discussion.

The second research question presented to students asked if they believed the electronic discussions enhanced their overall learning experience in this class (Table 2). Twenty-four (50%) of the students agreed or strongly agreed that the electronic discussion groups enhanced their learning experience, while 27% reported being neutral. Only 18 (38%) believed using keyboard pals enhanced their learning, while 11 (23%) stated they were neutral. When asked if these were appropriate learning tools, 77% reported that the electronic discussion group was an appropriate tool to use when covering diversity content. Only about half (52%) of the students felt the keyboard pals were an appropriate method to use.

The third research question related to students' comfort level with using technology after taking this course. Thirty-six (75%) students reported that using the electronic listserv improved their technology skills, while 15 (31%) students agreed or strongly agreed that using keyboard pals improved their technology skills. The students were also asked about their comfort level using technology in general after taking this course (Table 3). Students reported they felt very comfortable or comfortable (73%) with e-mail usage. They also felt very comfortable or comfortable (77%) with Internet use and with using the listserv (65%). Students also reported being very comfortable or comfortable (75%) with word processing.

TABLE 2. Student Perceptions Regarding Learning Experience–Frequency (Percentages) N = 48

Technology	Strongly Agree	Agree	Neutral	Disagree	Strongly Disagree
Electronic Group *(Enhanced learning?)*	10 (20.8)	14 (29.2)	13 (27.1)	7 (14.6)	3 (6.3)
Keyboard Pals *(Enhanced learning?)*	2 (4.2)	16 (33.3)	11 (23)	13 (27.1)	6 (12.5)
Electronic Group *(Appropriate tool?)*	15 (31.2)	22 (45.8)	6 (12.5)	1 (2.1)	2 (8.3)
Keyboard Pals *(Appropriate tool?)*	8 (16.7)	17 (35.4)	14 (29.2)	5 (10.4)	4 (8.3)

TABLE 3. Comfort with Technology–Frequency (Percentages) N = 48

Technology	Very Comfortable	Comfortable	Uncomfortable	Very Uncomfortable
Email	26 (54.2)	9 (18.8)	7 (14.6)	6 (12.5)
Internet	22 (48.8)	15 (31.3)	6 (12.5)	5 (10.4)
Listserv	17 (35.4)	14 (29.2)	10 (20.8)	7 (14.6)
Word Processing	28 (58.3)	8 (16.7)	5 (10.4)	7 (14.6)
TOTALS	48 (100)	48 (100)	48 (100)	48 (100)

Next, students were asked if they believed the use of computer mediated communications empowered students by giving them more responsibility for their own learning. Twenty-nine students (61%) agreed or strongly agreed that this learning experience was empowering. Last, when asked if the electronic group fostered a "sense of community" just over half (52%) of the students agreed or strongly agreed with this question. It should be noted that this question may have been ambiguous, as exemplified by the number of students who chose a neutral response (31%) for this question.

Narrative Comments

Many of the students offered narrative comments on the surveys, and several themes emerged. One of those themes was the idea that it gave everyone a chance to share opinions. One student stated, "it helped us to look further than we normally would to study other cultures, religions, etc. We all tend to get stuck in our own world and it was interesting to casually discuss others' interests and backgrounds." Students felt that they were able to be more honest on the listserv, and/or had more time to think about their reply before having to make a comment. Several of the students also expressed their wish that more students had been vocal, both in class and on the listserv.

Students overwhelmingly felt that the keyboard partners were not beneficial. The reasons given for this were mostly due to technical difficulties and/or lack of student interest. One student stated, "the keyboard pals was a waste of time because my partner would not respond to me. I felt stupid bringing up subjects that would get no response." Some were also uncomfortable with the idea of "talking" to someone they did not know. One student commented, "I really enjoyed the listserv but was uncomfortable with individual e-mail. It's hard being partnered with someone you really don't know." Some students suggested that if all keyboard pals had been interested in participating, this could have been a more profitable experience.

Most of the students who gave qualitative statements felt that the listserv was by far the best experience for them. Although students were frustrated with the technological glitches, they felt positive about their experiences overall. Some of the students also commented that the increased use of technology would be beneficial for their future educational and career prospects.

STUDENT RESPONSES ON LISTSERV

After deleting all duplicated and introductory messages, there were a total of 553 messages on the electronic board. Thirty-seven percent of the messages posted were about current events in the news that were not necessarily discussed in class. While there was 204 messages posted regarding current events in the news, only half (100) of them were specifically related to diversity content. For example, students wanted to discuss the school shooting at Columbine High School, the outbreak of war in Kosovo, and the impeachment proceedings of President Clinton. Although these messages were not related to the diversity class, they did reflect students' interest and concerns during the time this course was offered. The number of students who responded to current events that were more in tandem with the diversity course is listed in Table 4.

Students were also instructed to bring questions and various topics of interest to the electronic discussion group. This gave students an opportunity to discuss diversity issues that could not be covered in the classroom due to time constraints. There were 59 messages posted that fit the general category of outside diversity issues (Table 4).

Students seemed particularly interested in discussing relationships between people from different ethnic groups (Table 5). The majority of students defended the laws regarding desegregation in the school system, but few exemplified a true understanding of the complexity of this issue. Their comments suggested a certain naiveté regarding the history and legal issues related to desegregation. Many of the students also expressed surprise that interracial marriages were ever illegal in the United States, and most students defended this practice. The re-

TABLE 4

Current events related to diversity	Frequency
Texas court case–murder of African American man	22
KKK rallies in town and hate crimes	28
Racism among law enforcement	13
Teacher who made racist comment	9
Jim Crow Laws (started after program seen on TV)	8
Murder of gay man in Wyoming	8
Diversity training (in the news)	7
Opinion on the death penalty	5
Total	**100**
General questions/opinions related to diversity issues	
Can a woman be president?	18
General "live and let live" statements	16
Opinions on causes of prejudice or racism	8
Ability diversity	7
Why are there mostly women in social work?	7
Women in sports	6
Women as police officers	5
Corporate women "giving back" to community	5
Opinions about whether their schools were culturally biased	5
Opinions about whether social workers must be liberal	5
Should Internet be censured?	7
Should we ban talk shows?	6
Total	**95**

TABLE 5

Relationship Between People from Different Ethnic Groups	Frequency
Desegregation	37
Interracial marriages	32
Black children raised in White homes	15
Total	**84**

sponses were mixed regarding the practice of African American children being raised by White parents.

The remainder of the listserv comments were related to comments on classroom activity or readings (35), comments on specific ethnic groups (33), personal questions or shared experiences (28), and gay and lesbian issues (27). While nineteen responses dealt with religious beliefs and ideals directly, students' religious beliefs were sprinkled throughout many of their comments. This topic seemed to invoke the most passionate responses in students, who often disagreed about the role of religion in the social work profession.

APPLICATION TO SOCIAL WORK EDUCATION

Students were given very little direction for the electronic assignments other than to post at least 10 messages related to diversity on the listserv. We recommend that professors give students more specific instructions regarding the topics that should be discussed on the listserv, to help them stay focused on diversity issues. It is interesting to note how many of the posted messages were inspired by events that students read or heard about through the media. An unintended consequence of this type of assignment is that students are at least exposed to contemporary events, albeit through the filter of their peers' perceptions. This helped to make the topic of diversity more applicable to their own lives. Students spent little time rehashing class discussions but instead branched out to other areas. This certainly expanded the types and number of discussions that students were able to have with one another.

The instructors rarely offered their own opinions on the listserv because they wanted the students to feel a sense of "ownership" over their learning experience. Our hope was that students would feel more empowered regarding their learning in this class, and would not simply say what they thought the instructors wanted to hear. The students decided what direction the discussions would take.

In spite of technical problems experienced by students, and/or the amount of time spent learning to log on and utilize the listserv, most students felt this was a valuable experience. Although only 50 percent of students agreed that the electronic discussion group "enhanced their learning" in this class, the majority reported that the electronic discussions gave quieter students more opportunities to participate. Students also reported that they were able to bring up subjects on the listserv that they might not have brought up in class, and that they took more time to think about their responses than they do in traditional classroom discussions.

Overall, students believe they were given opportunities to discuss topics they felt were important, and hear from other students whose opinions might differ from their own. When students are participating in an electronic discussion, they are more likely to use good critical thinking skills as they reflect on what has been said rather than reacting simply on an emotional level. Sixty-one percent of the students reported that they found this experience to be empowering as they were given more responsibility for their own learning.

Due to the increased use of computers and online communication, practitioners need to be prepared to practice in the 21st century. It is incumbent on social work educators to help prepare students for this technology. E-mail and discussion groups are helpful ways to increase the comfort level of students with computers and their usage. "We have entered an information age in which power comes to those who have information and know how to access it" (Berge & Collins, 1995, p. 4). It is hoped that through these online opportunities, students will overcome the initial computer phobia that many students feel as they begin their coursework.

REFERENCES

Banks, R. E. & Coombs, N. (1995). *Your onramp to the internet: The power of electronic mail.* [On-line]. Available: *http://www.rit.edu/~nrcgsh/arts/aahebc95.html.*

Berge, Z.L., & Collins, M.P. (1995). *Introduction in computer mediated communication and the online classroom.* Cresskill, NJ: Hampton Press.

Council on Social Work Education (1994). Handbook of Accreditation Standards and Procedures. Washington, DC: Council on Social Work Education.

Edwards, S.L. (1998). Teaching Strategies for Multicultural Competence (Doctoral dissertation, University of South Carolina, 1997). *Dissertation Abstracts International*, 9815499.

Guernsey, L. (1997, Oct. 17). E-Mail is now used in a third of college courses. *The Chronicle of Higher Education.*

Hall, B. (1993). Using e-mail to enhance class participation. *Political Science & Politics*, *26* (4), 757-761.

Huff, M. T. (1998). *A comparison of critical thinking in an interactive television social work course.* (Doctoral dissertation, University of South Carolina, 1998.) *Dissertation Abstracts International*, 9815600.

Jackson, B., Yorker, B., & Mitchem, P. (1996). Teaching cultural diversity in a virtual classroom. *Journal of Child and Adolescent Psychiatric Nursing*, *9* (4), 40-43.

Karayan, S. & Crowe, J. (1997). Student perceptions of electronic discussion groups. *T.H.E. Journal: Technological Horizons in Education*, *24*(9), 69-71.

Latting, J.K. (1994). Diffusion of Computer-Mediated Communication in a Graduate Social Work Class: Lessons from "The Class from Hell." *Computers in Human Services*, *10*(3) 21-45.

Lewis, D., Treves, J.A. & Shaindlin, A.B. (1997). Making sense of academic cyberspace: Case study of an electronic classroom. *College Teaching*, *45*(3) 96-101.

Paul, R. W. (1990b). Dialogical thinking: Critical thought essential to the acquisition of rational knowledge and passions. In A. J. Binker (Ed.), *Critical thinking: What every person needs to survive in a rapidly changing world* (pp. 204-223). Rohnert Park, CA: Sonoma University.

Enhancing Critical Thinking and Professionalism Through Use of the Discussion Forum in Social Work Practice Courses

Janet L. Pray

SUMMARY. Development of critical thinking skills, application of theory, ethical decision-making, and achieving a professional identity are among the goals of social work education. This paper describes a three-year experience integrating discussion forums into graduate and undergraduate practice courses. Forums were designed to promote students' ability to use theory, analyze controversial issues, analyze and address ethical issues, professionally critique the work of peers, and conceptualize practice problems and issues for discussion in the forum. Evaluations indicated that discussion forums enhanced the depth of thinking about practice and practice issues and increased the sense of collegiality among students. *[Article copies available for a fee from The Haworth Document Delivery Service: 1-800-342-9678. E-mail address: <getinfo@haworthpressinc.com> Website: <http://www.HaworthPress.com> © 2001 by The Haworth Press, Inc. All rights reserved.]*

KEYWORDS. Technology, discussion forum, social work, critical thinking

---

Address correspondence to: Janet L. Pray, PhD, Professor and Chair, Department of Social Work, Gallaudet University, 800 Florida Avenue, NE, Washington, DC 20002-3695 (E-mail: Janet.Pray@gallaudet.edu).

The author wishes to thank Deirdre Mcglynn for her consultation and technical support which made this project possible.

[Haworth co-indexing entry note]: "Enhancing Critical Thinking and Professionalism Through Use of the Discussion Forum in Social Work Practice Courses." Pray, Janet L. Co-published simultaneously in *Journal of Technology in Human Services* (The Haworth Press, Inc.) Vol. 18, No. 1/2, 2001, pp. 65-75; and: *Using Technology in Human Services Education: Going the Distance* (ed: Goutham M. Menon, and Nancy K. Brown) The Haworth Press, Inc., 2001, pp. 65-75. Single or multiple copies of this article are available for a fee from The Haworth Document Delivery Service [1-800-342-9678, 9:00 a.m. - 5:00 p.m. (EST). E-mail address: getinfo@haworthpressinc.com].

An examination of the literature reveals a significant increase within the past few years in the use of technology in the interest of enhancing teaching and learning among many professions, including social work. The focus of much of the literature has been on using technology in the traditional classroom, using technology to support distance education, and preparing students for careers that appear destined to be increasingly technology dependent. Consider, for example, that forty-six of the 54 jobs identified by the U.S. Department of Labor as having the highest growth potential require skills in the use of technology (Rosenthal, 1999). There is evidence of growing interest among social work educators and practitioners in the potential for technology. Note, for example, presentations related to technology at the Annual Program Meetings of the Council on Social Work Education (CSWE) and National Association of Social Workers (NASW) conferences, two successful conferences sponsored by the College of Social Work at the University of South Carolina and a third one taking place September 1999. CSWE's Millennium Project provided funding to help support exploration of the use of technology in social work education. Currently most social work conferences include presentations devoted to some aspect of technology in education or practice.

Looking outside of social work, a recent article described the use of electronic communication tools for building collaborative learning communities for teaching organic chemistry (Glaser & Poole, 1999). Some proponents of total quality management are advocating the use of "electronic communities" for promoting the development of critical thinking skills (Miller, 1997). In the year 2000, the National Council for the Accreditation of Teacher Education (NCATE) will require accredited university programs to have faculty able to integrate technology into their courses as well as to prepare teachers who will use technology in their instruction (Rosenthal, 1999).

Some view the growth of technology as providing opportunities for educational innovation, for making educational programs available to those who otherwise might not have access, and for preparing students for the demands of jobs and careers in the 21st century. Others express concern that technology is depersonalizing education and creating distance between teachers and learners. With respect to this issue, an August 1998 article on the Web (Kearsley, 1998) provided an analysis of the characteristics of 184 courses from 148 institutions submitted to the Paul Allen Foundation Virtual Education contest that offered a

$25,000 prize for the most outstanding online course in higher education. The author's concluding statement notes that:

> . . . the most important overall impact of online courses is the emphasis they place on critical thinking and discourse. The one thing that happens in all online courses, regardless of the discipline or grade level, is that students communicate a lot more with each other and with the instructor. They discuss ideas, analyze, evaluate, argue, debate, and question. Online education redirects learning towards a constructivist and experiential mode on a large scale. This is a significant contribution of technology to improving our educational system. (Kearsley, 1998, p. 6)

Of particular interest in relation to the focus of this article is Kearsley's finding that among the submissions there was "little evidence that courses were designed to accommodate the needs of those with disabilities, which is especially a problem with courses that involve a lot of multimedia features" (Kearsley, 1998, p. 5). This finding among these proposals is in contrast to Gilbert's statement that, "Applications of information technology are now available that enable students and faculty–independent of most disabilities–to participate fully in all types of academic activities" (Gilbert, 1996, p. 47). This issue is of particular relevance to this article because approximately half of the students who participated in the discussion forums described herein are deaf or hard of hearing and some have other disabilities, including learning disabilities.

NATURE AND GOALS OF THE TECHNOLOGY PROJECT

The discussion forum was a key component of a project designed to incorporate technology into the social work curriculum at Gallaudet University in Washington, DC during a three-year period (1997 through 1999). During this time technology was integrated into graduate social work practice courses at the micro and macro levels in the Master's Program in Social Work, undergraduate Senior Seminar, MSW Field Seminar, graduate and undergraduate policy courses, and in research. Discussion forums were used in all of these courses. Classes during this three year period were comprised of a diverse group of students: deaf, hard of hearing, deaf with a learning disability, hard of hearing with a learning disability, hearing with a learning disability, and hearing students with no known disability. The decision to supplement traditional teaching methods with the use of computer technology was grounded in four major goals:

Empowering Learners. Technological resources such as Web-based discussion forums, various software programs, Internet sites, etc., provided opportunities to augment traditional instructional methods. Among the potential benefits are the ability to tailor teaching and learning to the needs of students with diverse learning styles and needs. A publication of the Gallaudet University Office for Students with Disabilities (1998) notes that, "students with learning disabilities feel easily overwhelmed in regular classes and struggle to keep up with the pace of the class . . . [and] may perform better [when] they can work at their own pace . . . " (p. 25). With this perspective in mind an asynchronous discussion forum was considered to be a good supplement to live discussions in the classroom, allowing students time to think through their contributions. An additional consideration is that deaf students learn through visual means and technology expands opportunities for deaf and other students who are visual learners.

For all students the opportunity to discuss case material in depth in a discussion forum (password protected to assure confidentiality) was seen as an additional way to promote application of theory, discuss approaches to complex issues related to values and ethics, and for students to develop skills in appropriate critiquing of each other's work. The discussion forum also offers opportunities for student initiated discussions. These student initiated discussions provide a means for addressing the needs of all students (particularly adult learners and non-traditional students) for recognition and appreciation of the value of their knowledge, experience, and perspectives.

Extending Resources. There are many resources available on the Web, including those specific to deafness, learning disabilities, and other disabilities. For example, there are journal articles from *The American Annals of the Deaf*, the *Journal of Deaf Studies and Deaf Education*, information from national and international deaf organizations, and support groups online. Availability of these and other resources on the Web enable students to search Web databases, conduct preliminary searches in some publications, obtain information from social work and other professional organizations, track legislation and communicate with legislators, identify client support and self-help groups, and bring the results of their explorations into the discussion forum.

Eliminating Barriers. Discussions in the traditional classroom favor students who are assertive, can formulate ideas quickly, and are comfortable speaking in a group. Shy students, students with certain types of disabilities, and students who need more time to organize their thinking are at a disadvantage during class discussions, many of which are fast-paced. As noted earlier, the asynchronous discussion forum allows students to take as much time as they need to formulate and think through their contributions. They also have an opportunity to edit their submission if the instructor sets the forum up to permit students to do so.

Enhancing Employability. With the use of technology on the rise in programs and agencies in the community, graduates with experience using technology often have a competitive edge in the marketplace. There are at least 7500 child welfare workers online in California and they were trained at considerable expense. As social workers need to be replaced or others added, the agencies employing them would not be eager to have to engage in expensive training of new staff in the use of technology. Although controversial and fraught with ethical and legal implications, there are also people seeking counseling and support online. There are increasing opportunities for continuing education and professional development online. Social workers who are comfortable with technology will have these additional resources available to help them remain current in the field and satisfy continuing education requirements for licensing.

THE DISCUSSION FORUM

The discussion forum used by Gallaudet University is part of Gallaudet Dynamic Online Collaboration (GDOC), an integrated system developed by Eduprise (formerly known as Collegis) and modified to meet the needs of Gallaudet's faculty, staff, and students. This system can be used to put course syllabi, library resources, lectures, assignments, examinations,Web links, and discussion forums online. All of these areas are linked, thus once a faculty member or student accesses the "course center," it is possible to connect to any of these areas. There is also a link to the University Library catalog and data bases such as Eric, Social Work Abstracts, and Psych Abstracts. The link to the University Library includes online access to the catalogs of all the university libraries in the Washington Resource Library Consortium. The course center may also be linked to Proquest, a service to which the University subscribes giving faculty and students access to journal articles online. Links can be created in the discussion forum to the Web sites of professional organizations such as The National Association of Social Workers, the Council on Social Work Education, The Association of Social Work Boards, the American Society for Deaf Children, and any others of the instructor's or student's choice. Assignments may be submitted online (privately) to the instructor. In addition to posting public entries in the discussion forum, students may send private e-mails to the instructor or to each other from within the forum. At the instructor's discretion, students may be permitted to initiate new topics. In the judgment and experience of the author, it is an indicator of the success of the forum when students are motivated to post topics in which they are interested. The GDOC system gives the instructor the ability to edit or delete any posting considered inappropriate. During the three years of the project it has never been necessary for an instructor to use this function.

The author has made extensive use of a discussion forum in graduate practice courses, advanced practice seminars, and in an undergraduate senior seminar. The specific uses of the forum have included the following:

Continuation/Expansion of Class Discussion. What practice instructor has not had a class end at the height of a "hot" discussion? Rarely is it possible to recapture the spirit of the discussion the next time the class meets. With the discussion forum students and instructor can continue the discussion online, often drawing more students into the discussion and deepening the level of the contributions. One objective for the forum is increased use of critical thinking and professionalism which the author believes may be fostered when students must put their points of view in writing for public view by their peers and the instructor.

Discussion/Critique of Case Presentations and Other Presentations. Initially the instructor gave assignments in the forum for students to critique presentations given by fellow students. Specific guidelines for the critique were provided by the instructor. Over time students began to find the structure of these assignments somewhat tedious. As a result, the structure was modified so that students and the instructor would raise questions or issues as they seemed relevant to particular presentations. Students then began to take greater ownership of the forum, initiating numerous penetrating questions and making cogent observations. An important characteristic of the students' participation was that they were almost invariably supportive of each other, pointing out strengths before posing a challenge or offering different points of view. The exception occurred in an undergraduate class where a student who was disliked by some classmates was treated dismissively in the forum by a couple of fellow students. The instructor addressed the issue within the context of the forum from the perspective of the professional behavior expected towards colleagues as set forth in the NASW Code of Ethics. The dismissive behavior diminished in the forum but, unfortunately, did not stop entirely.

Discussion Critique of Readings. There seems never to be sufficient time in class to cover the assigned readings adequately. Initially the instructor posed questions related to the readings for discussion in the forum. Soon thereafter students posed questions, addressed controversial issues from the readings, critiqued and sometimes challenged the authors of texts and journal articles.

Topics and Cases Developed by the Instructor for Student Response. These were developed to give students the opportunity to share their perspectives on management of particular kinds of practice situations and to critique in a constructive way the points of view of others. Examples of situations include how to respond to a deaf client who tells the hearing social worker that her signs are "fine," but shows by her responses that she was not understanding what the social worker was attempting to communicate.

Application of Theory to Case Situations. Students examine theories, discuss how they would manage a particular case situation, and discuss the theory or theories that support their approach. Students struggle the most with this kind of assignment because it requires specific and clear integration of theory with practice. Students will frequently have lengthy online discussions with each other about which is the "right" theory to use and whether particular approaches and techniques are consistent with the theory.

Identification of Ethical Issues in Practice and Application of Ethical Decision Making Models for Resolution of These Issues. There are lengthy and heated discussions in class which carry over to the discussion forum related to ethical and unethical professional behavior, competing values and the relative merit of hierarchies of values that have been developed, limits on confidentiality, and ethical decision-making models. In one advanced practice class, several students took the initiative to search the literature for alternative models for resolving ethical dilemmas and introduced into the forum discussion about what they found.

Student Initiated Discussion of Practice Issues. Students bring to the forum for discussion issues that they have concern about, which range from identifying the role school social workers could have in the aftermath of Littleton, Colorado, pursuing issues that have arisen in other classes and about which they do not have closure, and the amount of self-disclosure that is appropriate when working with an adolescent.

Student Initiated Discussion of Issues, Problems, etc., from Their Field Practica. Students will frequently use the discussion forum to solicit the points of view of other students about issues they are dealing with in their field practicum. These include concerns that a client is not receiving all the services to which he is entitled, questions of ethical/unethical behavior on the part of a colleague, questions/concerns about one's role as a social work intern, collaborating with interns from other disciplines, identification of problems in the field practicum agency, and innumerable other issues.

EVALUATION OF DISCUSSION FORUM USE

MSW Students. Each semester students anonymously evaluate the course and instructor. They are also asked to do a separate, anonymous evaluation of the use of technology in the course, including the discussion forum. The vast majority of students have been consistently positive about the ways in which they perceive the discussion forum to have enhanced their learning and their development as professionals. During the second semester of a practice class the students asked whether a forum could be set up for them to use for peer support and consultation after receiving their MSW degree. They expressed appreciation for each other and the ways in which they supported each other's learning in a constructive way, even when they were not in agreement. Ultimately, they set up a forum ("Deaf, hard of hearing, and hearing social workers") as a project for another class and have opened it up to social workers throughout the country and internationally who work with deaf and hard of hearing people. Participation in the forum waned dramatically after students received their degrees but with faculty promotion of the forum, persistence of one of the graduates, and postings of employment opportunities, forum participation began to increase.

The aspect of the forum which MSW students found most useful was the discussions students initiated themselves. They also were highly favorable about how comfortable they were risking being open in the discussion forum, feeling that the key factor was their trust in each other and in the instructor.

Two criticisms of the forum were that students felt that they put a great deal more effort and time into the practice courses with a discussion forum than in courses without a forum. They viewed the forum as providing additional work without reducing any of the other expectations for the course. They also felt that as other instructors have become interested in using discussion forums they began to have to spend too much time in the forums and that some overlapped in purpose. Cited as an example was the author's discussion forum for the Advanced Practice Seminar and the forum for the Field Practicum Seminar. As a result of that feedback the two forums will be combined into one and the two instructors will participate jointly in the one forum. This seemed a logical resolution, and perhaps an improvement, because of the close relationship between practice and field practicum.

Undergraduate Students. During the three year period there was just one undergraduate class taught by this instructor using a discussion forum. The students rated the forum highly and a number commented that their online discussions made them feel more professional than when they were discussing similar issues in class. Seniors also initiated their own discussion topics as the semester progressed, but their participation in the forum was never as extensive as the MSW students. The class requested a discussion in the forum of a problem they were having with another class. Initially students primarily ventilated their frustration, but as the semester progressed they used the forum to brainstorm solutions. At the conclusion of the course they requested that the entire forum be erased because of their concerns about the sensitive nature of the discussion they had about the other course. Their request was honored and the forum was deleted at the end of the semester.

DISCUSSION

Although there are no data to show cause and effect and although there are variables to be taken into account other than use/non-use of a discussion forum, it is interesting to note that the grades for students in the MSW practice courses taught by the author are significantly higher than they were before forum use. The author's observation is that most graduate students invest considerable amounts of time in the forum and the more they use the forum, the more professionally sophisticated their contributions to discussions become. During the 1998-1999 academic year the graduate students were delving extensively into practice issues and on their own initiative brought readings to the discussion–not only required readings, but readings they had done on their own. They also provided extensive support to each other and gave sophisticated feedback about their practice.

In one of the graduate courses a small number of deaf students expressed concern about participating in the discussion forum because English was their second language. They were referring to American Sign Language (ASL) as their first language and had concern that their written English was not as good as hearing classmates whose first language was English. They were asked to give the forum a try and were told that the requirement for participating could be reviewed if they continued to feel uncomfortable. The issue was not raised again by any deaf students in that class and the students who had expressed the concern participated as actively as the rest of the class.

All but one of the undergraduate students in the Senior Seminar participated regularly as required for the course. One student took the initiative for identifying Web sites related to issues being discussed in class and in the forum and he created some links to those sites. Another student raised an ethical issue she wanted the class to discuss online and most of the students made appropriate but brief comments. There needs to be more experience with undergraduate students majoring in social work before drawing any firm conclusions about the value of forum use. Comparing just this one class with the MSW students, it was clear that the MSW students experienced the discussion forum as far more meaningful to their learning than the undergraduate students did.

Based upon a three-year experience, student evaluations, and personal observation, it appears that use of a discussion forum does have potential for enhancing the development of critical thinking skills and professional behavior among students, particularly graduate students.

REFERENCES

Gilbert, S.W. (1996). Making the most of a slow revolution. *Change: The Magazine of Higher Learning 28* (2), 10-23.

Glaser, R. E. & Pool, M. J. (1999). Organic chemistry online: Building collaborative learning communities through electronic communication tools. *Journal of Chemical Education 76* (5), 699-703.

Kearsley, G. (1998 August). Online education: New paradigms for learning and teaching [On-line]. Available: http://horizon.unc.edu/TS/vision/, 1-7.

Miller, L. R. (1997). Better ways to think and communicate. *Association Management 49* (13), 71-73.

Office of Students with Disabilities (1998). *The Gallaudet Learning Disabilities Handbook.*

Rosenthal, I.G. & Poftak, A. (1999). New teachers and technology: Are they prepared? *Technology and Learning 19*, 22-24.

Distance Education: The Role of the Site Advisory Committee

Christine B. Kleinpeter
Marilyn K. Potts
John Oliver

SUMMARY. This paper describes the role of the Site Advisory Committee (SAC) as a link between the off-campus sites and the host university. The role of the SAC is to provide advice, regional perspectives, and suggestions for distance education program enhancement. SAC activities, structure, and a program evaluation plan will be addressed. *[Article copies available for a fee from The Haworth Document Delivery Service: 1-800-342-9678. E-mail address: <getinfo@haworthpressinc.com> Website: <http://www.HaworthPress.com> © 2001 by The Haworth Press, Inc. All rights reserved.]*

KEYWORDS. Distance education, site advisory committee, DE site involvement

This paper describes the role of the Site Advisory Committee (SAC) in a three-year, part-time MSW Distance Education (DE) program. The program goals are to increase the number of rural graduated

Christine B. Kleinpeter is Assistant Professor, Marilyn K. Potts is Professor, and John Oliver is Director, Department of Social Work, California State University, 1250 Bellflower Blvd., Long Beach, CA 90840-0902.

Address correspondence to: Christine B. Kleinpeter.

An earlier version of this paper was presented at The Third Annual Technology Conference for Social Work Education and Practice.

[Haworth co-indexing entry note]: "Distance Education: The Role of the Site Advisory Committee." Kleinpeter, Christine B., Marilyn K. Potts, and John Oliver. Co-published simultaneously in *Journal of Technology in Human Services* (The Haworth Press, Inc.) Vol. 18, No. 1/2, 2001, pp. 77-87; and: *Using Technology in Human Services Education: Going the Distance* (ed: Goutham M. Menon, and Nancy K. Brown) The Haworth Press, Inc., 2001, pp. 77-87. Single or multiple copies of this article are available for a fee from The Haworth Document Delivery Service [1-800-342-9678, 9:00 a.m. - 5:00 p.m. (EST). E-mail address: getinfo@haworthpressinc.com].

educated social workers and to facilitate the development of MSW programs at rural universities. The present program model links eighty students at four rural sites using Interactive Television (ITV) to an urban host site, with on-site and off-site administration and instruction.

According to a 1996 survey, 16% of social work education programs reported the use of DE technology, a 5% increase over the previous two years (Siegal, Jennings, Conklin, & Napoletano Flynn, 1998). Conklin (1993) reviewed over 200 articles and concluded that no evidence existed to suggest that social work educators should not use DE technology. Empirical data indicate that the educational experiences and/or achievements of DE students are at least comparable to those of traditionally enrolled students (Forester, 1997; Haagenstad & Kraft, 1998; Haga & Heitkamp, 1995; Hollister & McGee, 1998; Perracchi & Patchner, 1998; Raymond, 1998). Results from DE student evaluations also indicate satisfaction levels at least equivalent to those obtained in traditional classrooms (Haga & Heitkamp, 1995; Jennings, Siegal & Conklin, 1995; Kikuchi & Sorensen, 1997).

However, there is concern regarding the professional socialization of DE students because of the lack of face-to-face contact with instructors (Olcott, Jr. & Wright, 1995). Horner and Whitbeck (1991) compared the values of social work students and faculty to the general population and found that social workers distinguish themselves from the general population in the importance they assign interpersonal relationships, service to others, open-mindedness, and self-concept.

Haga and Heitkamp (1995) reported that socialization for DE students occurs by the use of assistant instructors, site visits by course instructors, and presentations made over ITV by local NASW representatives. However, using a similar program model, Potts, Hagan, and Wilson (1998) found that the on-campus students saw the faculty as a reference group significantly more than did the DE students.

In the present program model, the SAC will be considered as both a reference group for students and as a link between the off-campus sites and the host university. The role of the SAC is to provide advice, regional perspectives, and suggestions for program enhancement (Tropman, Johnson, & Tropman, 1979). The goals of the SAC are to identify supplemental educational opportunities for students, to create linkages with the local health and human services agencies, to provide professional socialization activities for students, to encourage alumni involvement, and to assess the local needs for additional MSW professionals. The composition of the SAC includes the site coordinator; university administrators and faculty from the local site; alumni; students; and representatives from health and human services, county agencies, NASW, and the continuing education department of the local university. Suggested activities for the SAC include sponsoring professional socialization activities, identifying potential field placement sites/field instructors, planning alumni events, and providing information and suggestions for resolving program/system problems.

THE SITE ADVISORY COMMITTEE GUIDELINES

The guidelines for the SAC were developed by the Distance Education Committee, which consists of faculty and administrators from the Department of Social Work at the host university. The guidelines were developed using the KNOWER system (Tropman, 1984, cited in Tropman, 1997). The KNOWER system is a planning tool, which can be used for writing drafts and documents for community groups. The Distance Education Committee outlined the principles to be incorporated into the guidelines for the SAC as follows: goals and objectives, committee composition, structure and process, suggested activities, and line of communication. These principles were drafted into a first outline. The outline was presented to all committee members and to the site coordinators for feedback. The recommendations were incorporated into the second draft and taken to the Distance Education Committee for additional changes. The second draft was presented to the full faculty for feedback and recommendations. These recommendations were incorporated into the guidelines and the third draft was accepted by the faculty in January 1999 (Appendix 1).

DEVELOPMENT OF THE SITE ADVISORY COMMITTEES

The development of the SAC has varied across the four sites. Two of the sites have alumni as this is the second cohort in those communities, and two of the sites are new this year. At each of the continuing sites, there has been an alumni activity during the past year. At one site, the alumni met for a potluck dinner in the home of an alumnus and had a visiting professor and site coordinator update them on the changes in the program, as well as to ask them for input for future alumni activities. Alumni identified continuing education as an important aspect of future events, due to state licensing board requirements for continuing education. Most of the attending alumni identified "having an opportunity to network with colleagues" as an important aspect of the alumni functions. At this rural site there are 11 active members of the SAC including: local BSW faculty, the Chair of the local BSW program, the Director of Extended Education, members of the professional community, a technology consultant, current student representatives, and an alumni representative.

In the second community, the alumni were invited to meet with new students at a dinner held during the first month of the second cycle of the program. A visiting professor and the site coordinator met with both new students and alumni at a local restaurant. The alumni offered the new students a valuable perspective on how to succeed in the DE program. Some of the alumni offered to serve as mentors to the new students. In this community, the SAC meetings are held in conjunction with the local NASW chapter meetings. This rural community has 7-8 members who are active participants. The participants include members of the local professional community, faculty from the local BSW program, the present chair of the local BSW program, current student representatives, and an alumni representative.

The third community is actively working toward the opening of their own MSW program. The DE program at that site is used as a springboard for the opening of the new program. The SAC has met primarily to provide recommendations for the new program. Additionally, this committee has served the DE program by offering suggestions for field placement sites and supervisors, as well as identifying potential adjunct faculty.

The fourth community is currently forming its SAC. The site coordinator is actively identifying potential committee members. Currently, the site coordinator has met primarily with the Director of Social Services to assist with field placements for the new MSW class. This site currently has no plans for the development of an MSW program. The goal for this community is to meet the needs for additional social workers using DE. Therefore, the goal is to identify key members in the community who can serve as a more permanent link to the host university.

THE BENEFITS OF THE SITE ADVISORY COMMITTEES

The SACs have benefited the DE program in several ways, including recruitment of new students, identifying and providing professional socialization activities, and identifying potential field placement sites, as well as supervisors. The SAC has assisted the program by providing options for problem solving such as ordering books, connecting students with student services at the local sites, and coordination of graduation activities. Additionally, the SAC assesses the community needs for additional MSWs and makes recommendations for long-range planning. In both of our continuing sites, there is interest from the SAC in developing an MSW program in the local community. Both communities are currently assessing the need and resources available for this goal. The SAC will be helpful in this regard. As the host institution withdraws its involvement, the SACs will become a valuable resource to the new MSW programs.

POTENTIAL RISKS OF THE SITE ADVISORY COMMITTEES

Tropman et al. (1979) have outlined three procedural difficulties with advisory committees. These include: (1) "matters to be considered by the committee; (2) the relationship between the committee and the executive it is assisting; and (3) the matter or form in which the advice is to be presented" (p. 155). They recommend that the agenda be formulated by the chair of the committee in consultation with the executive group being advised. In this manner, the committee will be clear on what issues the executive group needs recommendations. However, it is noted that most advisory committees initiate advice as well as respond to requests for it. Tropman et al. (1979) recommended that minutes of the advisory committee meetings be given to the advisee. Additionally, they stated that sometimes it is helpful for the advisees to meet with the advisory committee in order for informal interaction and a fuller discussion of the issues.

Addressing the potential risks of advisory committees, Tropman et al. (1979) stated, "These committees are among the most common, and, in our experience, work on them is more subject to disillusionment and more frustrating than on almost any other type of committee" (p. 160). These authors point to the importance of keeping the group focused on its mission–to provide recommendations–as a key to avoiding disillusionment. They stress the need for the chair of the advisory committee to keep a balance between discussion and decision. Strong leadership was identified as the key to keeping the group on task and providing the feedback loop from the advisory committee to the advisee and from the executive group back to the committee.

Given the developmental nature of the DE program, it has not been difficult to maintain a focused approach for the SACs. If their role begins to wane as the program becomes more institutionalized, there may be an increase in disharmony and lack of task-directed focus.

DISCUSSION

The program described is now in its second cycle of the 3-year, part-time MSW program. The program has expanded from two remote sites to four. The students in the second cohort have doubled to nearly eighty. The SAC guidelines were requested by one of the original sites due to a lack of clarity regarding their purpose and mission. The frustrations which Tropman et al. (1979) described were reported, at times, by the SAC particularly when recommendations were not adopted by faculty at the host site. Additionally, the line of communication between the SAC and the faculty/administration at the host site was not clearly defined. This resulted in a perception that issues that were raised by the SAC were not being fully addressed by the host site. The formalizing of the line of communication, and the addition of a Director of Distance Education as a channel for communication between the site coordinators and the host site has been helpful in this regard.

Despite the potential risks inherent in advisory committees, the benefits far outweigh the risks for enhancement of the DE program. The SAC is in the unique position to inform the host site regarding the norms and practice standards in the off-campus sites; they are uniquely qualified and are experts on identifying and framing issues from a local perspective; they are an invaluable means of legitimizing and facilitating local ownership of the DE program; they contribute to the overall quality of professional social work by integrating the interest of diverse settings in a cooperative body; they understand the resources and limitations available at the remote locations; and they are in a position to provide an ongoing professional reference group for both current students and alumni.

LESSONS LEARNED

SACs are an important component of distance education. They provide the linkage between the university sponsoring the program, the host site, and the local practice community.

A variety of lessons were learned as a consequence of graduating one class from the DE program. Additional insights have been developed which are associated with challenges involved with doubling the size of the second cohort of distance education students. Among the lessons learned are:

- DE programs should develop an SAC policy document with input from departmental faculty, site coordinators, and relevant administrative personnel from the host campus (i.e., Deans of continuing education, technology, student services). This document should be made available to all stakeholders who are involved in the collaborative educational enterprise. The involvement of stakeholders will be of assistance in developing broad-based host and practice community committee representation, assist in developing a perception of being able to influence the program at the local level, and help to develop the infrastructure needed to market and garner program support from the local human service community.
- Early and ongoing efforts must be made by the departmental program sponsors to facilitate empowerment of the SAC. In retrospect, it is clear that SAC members would benefit from receiving select faculty correspondence, faculty agendas plus attachments, and participation in a faculty meeting or DE committee meetings via use of the technology. These opportunities would be of assistance in mainstreaming faculty and SAC relationships by signaling their importance and value to the department.
- In addition to sharing departmental brochures and specialized publications with the SAC, an SAC handbook should be developed that clearly specifies SAC policy, roles, scope of authority, method of communication, and expectations. Preparation of such a document will assist the committee in planning activities that adhere to the parameters of SAC policy, and help them to retain the focus needed to complete appropriate activities and tasks effectively.

- The volume and spacing of planned SAC events were found to be directly related to the morale of group membership, their level of commitment to the program, and the quality of their involvement. Consequently, in addition to regularly scheduled meetings, it is also advisable that the SAC exercise leadership in developing events that current students, alumni, and local practitioners associate with their functions.

EVALUATION PLAN

Program evaluation will occur in three ways: (1) a content analysis of the SAC meetings to document the activities/suggestions provided; (2) attendance at the SAC meetings and professional socialization activities offered; and (3) qualitative interviews of the SAC members, selected students, and alumni regarding the extent to which they were satisfied with the function and process of the committee and the activities provided.

REFERENCES

Conklin, J. J. (1993). The development of a strategic plan for implementing distance education in social work education. (ERIC Document Reproduction Service No. ED 360 892).

Forester, M. (1997). Evaluating a part-time graduate social work distance education program at the University of Southern Mississippi. Paper presented at the Conference on Information Technologies for Social Work Education, Charleston, SC.

Haagenstad, S., & Kraft, S. (1998). Outcome measures comparing classroom education to distance education. Paper presented at the Conference on Information Technologies for Social Work Education and Practice, Charleston, SC.

Haga, M., & Heitkamp, T. L. (1995). Evaluation results of an innovative social work distance education program. Paper presented at the Annual Program Meeting of the Council on Social Work Education, San Diego, CA.

Hollister, C.D., & McGee, G. (1998). Delivering substance abuse and child welfare content through interactive television. Paper presented at the Conference on Information Technologies for Social Work Education and Practice, Charleston, SC.

Horner, W.C., & Whitbeck, L.B. (1991). Personal versus professional values in social work: A methodological note. *Journal of Social Service Research*, *14*(1/2), 21-43.

Jennings, J., Siegel, E., & Conklin, J.J. (1995). Social work education and distance learning: Applications for continuing education. *Journal of Continuing Social Work Education*, *6*, 3-7.

Kikuchi, S.L., & Sorensen, S.R. (1997). Reach out and touch someone: Experiences of the rural off-campus MSW program, Graduate School of Social Work, University of Utah. Paper presented at the Conference on Information Technologies of Social Work Education, Charleston, SC.

Olcott, D., & Wright, S.J. (1995). An institutional support framework for increasing faculty participation in postsecondary distance education. *The American Journal of Distance Education 9* (3), 5-17.

Patracchi, H.E., & Patchner, M.A. (1998). ITV versus face-to-face instruction: Outcomes of a two-year study. Paper presented at the Conference on Information Technologies for Social Work Education and Practice, Charleston, SC.

Potts, M.K., Hagan, C.B., & Wilson, G.K. (1998). A systems model of a distance education program: Input, throughput, output. Paper presented at the Annual Program Meeting of the Council on Social Work Education, Orlando, FL.

Raymond, F.B. (1998). Providing social work education and training in rural areas through interactive television. (ERIC Document Reproduction Services No. 309 910).

Siegel, E., Jennings, J.G., Conklin, J., & Napoletano Flynn, S.A. (1998). Distance learning in social work education: Results and implications of a national study. *Journal of Social Work Education*, *34*, 71-80.

Tropman, J.E., Johnson, H.R., & Tropman, E.J. (1979). *The Essentials of Committee Management*. Chicago, IL: Nelson-Hall.

Tropman, J.E. (1997). *Successful Community Leadership: A Skills Guide for Volunteers and Professionals*. Washington, DC: NASW Press Inc.

APPENDIX 1
Distance Education Advisory Committee Guidelines

The role of the Distance Education Advisory Committee is to provide advice, regional perspectives, and suggestions for program enhancement to the CSULB Department of Social Work Faculty, the decision-making body. Committee input and suggestions are an essential component in representing the unique needs and opportunities of each community.

Area 1–Goals and Objectives of the Distance Education Advisory Committees

- To identify supplemental educational opportunities for students
- To create linkages with the local health and human services agencies
- To provide general support for the MSW program objectives
- To participate in local macro-system problem solving
- To encourage active alumni involvement
- To serve as a resource for local educational and professional service needs
- To assess the local needs for additional MSW level professionals
- To provide input into student and agency recruitment
- To offer suggestions for program enhancement

Area 2–Distance Education Advisory Committee Suggested Composition (in addition to the ex-officio members: the Director of Distance Education and the Site Coordinator)

- University administrators and faculty (BSW or related disciplines)
- CSULB, Department of Social Work Alumni
- Current student representation
- Health and human services agency representatives
- County agencies (i.e., probation, child welfare, school district, and health)
- NASW representatives
- Continuing education representative

Area 3–Distance Education Advisory Committee Structure and Process

It is vital that each committee retain sufficient latitude to determine a structure and operating procedures compatible with its membership, constituents and community norms. To ensure continuity we recommend regularly scheduled meetings, election of officers, and development of a permanent record by recording and forwarding minutes to the CSULB, Department of Social Work Distance Education Office.

Area 4–Suggested Activities

- To sponsor professional socialization activities
- To assist in identifying appropriate field placement sites and potential field instructors
- To assist in identifying community that would be useful for student thesis research or community projects
- To assist in planning graduation activities
- To plan alumni events
- To provide information and suggestions to the site coordinator in resolving program/system problems
- To host supplemental educational activities relevant to the local site interests
- To provide networking opportunities for social work professionals and MSW students
- To establish ad hoc task groups as needed

Area 5–Line of Communication

The line of communication between the Distance Education Advisory Committee and CSULB Department of Social Work is carried from the Site Coordinator to the Director of Distance Education who will carry the information to the CSULB Department of Social Work Distance Education Committee and the appropriate CSULB department/person. The Distance Education Director will be responsible for communicating directly with the local Advisory Committees through the site coordinator.

Evaluating ITV-Based MSW Programs: A Comparison of ITV and Traditional Graduates' Perceptions of MSW Program Qualities

C. David Hollister
Youngmin Kim

SUMMARY. Traditional and ITV-based MSW graduates at the University of Minnesota are compared on their perceptions of learning, relationships with instructors, adequacy of access to resources, connections with others students, staff support, connection to the school. Possible impacts of ITV exposure on graduates' use of electronic technologies are also examined. ITV graduates generally rated the program's impacts on learning and their satisfaction with various program supports equal to or higher than did graduates of the traditional program, with the exception of students' connections to other students and access to resources such as libraries and computer labs. *[Article copies available for a fee from The Haworth Document Delivery Service: 1-800-342-9678. E-mail address: <getinfo@haworthpressinc.com> Website: <http://www.HaworthPress.com> © 2001 by The Haworth Press, Inc. All rights reserved.]*

C. David Hollister, PhD, is Professor at the University of Minnesota School of Social Work.

Youngmin Kim, MSW, is Research Assistant and a doctoral student at the University of Minnesota School of Social Work.

Correspondence may be addressed to the authors at: School of Social Work, University of Minnesota, 105 Peters Hall, 1404 Gortner Avenue, St. Paul, MN 55108.

[Haworth co-indexing entry note]: "Evaluating ITV-Based MSW Programs: A Comparison of ITV and Traditional Graduates' Perceptions of MSW Program Qualities." Hollister, C. David, and Youngmin Kim. Co-published simultaneously in *Journal of Technology in Human Services* (The Haworth Press, Inc.) Vol. 18, No. 1/2, 2001, pp. 89-100; and: *Using Technology in Human Services Education: Going the Distance* (ed: Goutham M. Menon, and Nancy K. Brown) The Haworth Press, Inc., 2001, pp. 89-100. Single or multiple copies of this article are available for a fee from The Haworth Document Delivery Service [1-800-342-9678, 9:00 a.m. - 5:00 p.m. (EST). E-mail address: getinfo@haworthpressinc.com].

KEYWORDS. Distance learning, interactive television, MSW programs, social work graduates, instructional support

A number of studies have evaluated individual social work courses taught at a distance (Rooney, Freddolino, Hollister, & Macy, 1999), but there is still a dearth of studies evaluating distance MSW programs as a whole. While there is evidence to suggest that learning outcomes in distance programs are comparable to traditional programs (Rooney et al., 1999), there remain many questions as to the qualities that are important for facilitating learning in distance versus traditional formats. For example, how much staff support is required? To what extent do students feel connected with the school offering the program, with the instructors, and with other students? How adequate is student access to resources such as libraries, computer labs, reserve readings, etc.? It is important to note at the outset that these questions are as appropriate to ask of traditional formats as of distance formats, in that traditional programs also vary in the adequacy of their solutions to these needs.

In addition to the above questions, the authors were interested to know whether the greater exposure to instructional technology experienced by graduates of the distance MSW program might result in their greater adoption of various electronic technologies, both while in graduate school and after graduation, compared to graduates of the traditional program. Is there a spillover effect?

Graduates' perceptions of their educational experiences can provide important data for faculty and administrators about program qualities, even though such perceptions must be considered alongside other measures and are only one part of the evaluation of a program.

The present study attempts to explore some of these questions by comparing the perceptions and experiences of recent graduates of the traditional and distance versions of the MSW program at the University of Minnesota School of Social Work. The School, located in the Twin Cities of Minneapolis/St. Paul, has offered an advanced standing, direct practice concentration by interactive television (ITV) to several remote sites since 1994 (Kalke, Rooney, & Macy, 1998).

METHODS

The subjects in this study were persons who had completed the MSW program at the University of Minnesota, Twin Cities anytime during 1998. Questions concerning the adequacy of various aspects of program support and the impact of the ITV format on learning and on graduates' use of technology were included in a questionnaire sent to all 1998 MSW graduates (N = 100) in February 1999. Sixty-seven questionnaires were returned by July 1999 (a 67% response rate).

In order to compare ITV and traditional graduates' perceptions, three categories of graduates were identified according to the proportion of ITV courses taken as part of the MSW program:

- Full-ITV graduates, who took the majority or all of their MSW coursework via ITV.
- Partial-ITV graduates, who took part of their MSW coursework via ITV.
- Traditional graduates, who took no MSW coursework via ITV.

As shown in Table 1, over sixty percent (n = 42) of the survey respondents took at least one ITV course during the MSW program. Of these, fifteen respondents completed their entire MSW coursework via ITV, while twenty-five (37.3%) took no ITV courses.

All of the full-ITV graduates and 19 of the 27 partial-ITV graduates (70.4%) were weekend students, while 24 out of 25 traditional graduates were weekday students. (See Table 2.) Weekend students take their courses on Friday evenings, Saturdays, and Sundays.

Among the full-ITV graduates who had been weekend students, twelve graduates (80.0%) completed the MSW program in Moorhead, two graduates (13.3%) completed it in Rochester, while one graduate completed the MSW program in the Twin Cities. All of the partial-ITV and traditional weekend graduates completed the MSW program in the Twin Cities. (See Table 3.)

TABLE 1. Distribution of the Respondents by Exposure to ITV Courses

Category	Frequency (n)	Percent (%)
Full-ITV graduates	15	22.4
Partial-ITV graduates	27	40.3
Traditional graduates	25	37.3
Total	67	100.0

DIMENSIONS OF PROGRAM SUPPORT

The above three categories of graduates were compared on their perceptions of the extent to which the program supported their studies. Graduates were asked to rate the following characteristics of the MSW program:

- Staff support for students;
- Students' connection with the school;
- Students' relationships with instructors;
- Adequacy of access to resources, e.g., library, copying, computer labs;
- Students' connections to other students;
- Access to relevant course materials; and
- Site coordination and support (asked of distance students only).

Graduates were asked to rate each item as follows: 1 = poor, 2 = needs improvement, 3 = satisfactory, 4 = good, 5 = excellent. The mean score for each item was compared among the three categories of graduates, as shown in Table 4.

TABLE 2. Distribution of Respondents in Program Tracks

Status	Full-ITV	Partial-ITV	Traditional	Total
Weekend	15 (100%)	19 (70.4%)	1 (4.0%)	35 (52.2%)
Weekday	0	8 (29.6%)	24 (96.0%)	32 (47.8%)

TABLE 3. Location of Weekend Students (n = 34*)

Location	Full-ITV	Partial-ITV*	Traditional
Moorhead	12 (80.0%)	0	0
Rochester	2 (13.3%)	0	0
Twin Cities	1 (6.7%)	18 (100%)	1 (100%)
Total	15 (100%)	18 (100%)	1 (100%)

* Missing data = 1.

Full-ITV graduates rated site coordination and support very highly. They also rated the other items *higher* than did traditional graduates, with the exceptions of adequacy of access to resources, $F(2, 63) = 5.62, p < .01$, and students' connections to other students, $F(2, 63) = 0.96, p > .05$. Full-ITV graduates also expressed higher satisfaction on two items, access to relevant course materials, $F(2, 63) = 8.04, p = .001$, and staff support for students, $F(2, 63) = 2.51, p > .05$, than did either traditional or partial-ITV graduates, although the differences in staff support for students did not reach statistical significance. Curiously, partial-ITV graduates expressed the highest satisfaction on students' connection to the school, $F(2, 63) = 4.72, p < .05$, and students' relationships with instructors, $F(2, 62) = 1.14, p > .05$.

TABLE 4. Graduates' Satisfaction with Program Support

Items*	Full-ITV n = 15	Partial-ITV n = 27	Traditional n = 24**	Grand means n = 66***	Oneway ANOVA	
					F	*p*
Staff support for students	3.67 (0.98)	3.30 (1.03)	2.92 (1.06)	3.24 (1.05)	2.51	.089
Students' connection to the school	2.53 (0.74)	3.07 (0.68)	2.50 (0.78)	2.74 (0.77)	4.72	.012
Students' relationships with instructors	3.33 (0.62)	3.63 (0.74)	3.30 (1.02)	3.45 (0.83)	1.14	.327
Adequacy of access to resources	2.93 (0.80)	2.70 (0.87)	3.50 (0.88)	3.05 (0.92)	5.62	.006
Students' connections to other students	3.47 (0.74)	3.41 (0.89)	3.75 (1.03)	3.55 (0.91)	0.96	.387
Access to relevant course materials	3.93 (0.80)	2.96 (0.76)	3.63 (0.88)	3.42 (0.90)	8.04	.001
Site coordination and support	4.47 (0.74)	N.A.	N.A.	N.A.	N.A.	

* Possible ratings were 1 = poor; 2 = needs improvement; 3 = satisfactory; 4 = good; 5 = excellent.
** n = 24, except students' relationships with instructor (n = 23).
*** n = 66 except students' relationships with instructor (n = 65).
( ) = S. D.

PERCEIVED IMPACT OF ITV ON LEARNING

Full-ITV graduates and partial-ITV graduates were asked whether ITV courses enhanced or hindered their learning. The questionnaire asked: "When you compare the ITV courses to more traditional classroom courses you have taken in the past, did the delivery of the ITV courses: (1) enhance your learning very much, (2) enhance your learning somewhat, (3) make no difference in your learning, (4) hinder your learning somewhat, or (5) hinder your learning very much."

As shown in Table 5, over two-thirds of the full-ITV graduates said that ITV instruction either made no difference to their learning or enhanced their learning. Only four indicated that ITV hindered their learning somewhat, and none said that it hindered learning very much. The partial-ITV graduates were more mixed in their responses with only half indicating either that ITV made no difference or that it enhanced their learning. Likewise, in Table 5 the mean rating (3.29) of partial-ITV graduates is somewhat less favorable toward ITV instruction than is the mean rating (2.79) of the full-ITV graduates. However, this difference is not statistically significant, $t = -1.248, p > .05$.

TABLE 5. Comparison of ITV Courses to Traditional Courses by Full- and Partial-ITV Graduates

	Full-ITV Graduates	Partial-ITV Graduates
ITV enhanced learning very much	2 (14.3%)	1 (7.1%)
ITV enhanced learning somewhat	3 (21.4%)	2 (14.3%)
ITV made no difference	5 (35.7%)	4 (28.6%)
ITV hindered learning somewhat	4 (28.6%)	6 (42.9%)
ITV hindered learning very much	0	1 (7.1%)
Total**	14 (100.0%)	14 (100.0%)
Mean (S. D.)***	2.79 (1.05)	3.29 (1.07)

* Possible ratings were 1 = enhance learning very much; 2 = enhance learning somewhat; 3 = make no difference; 4 = hinder learning somewhat; 5 = hinder learning very much.

** x^2 (4, 28) = 2.044, p = .728

*** t (26) = −1.248, p = .223

PERCEIVED IMPACT OF ITV COURSES ON USE OF TECHNOLOGY

It is conceivable that exposure to ITV technology could have an effect of stimulating ITV graduates' adoption of newer technologies in other aspects of their work, a so-called "spillover" effect, in that instructors of ITV courses usually encouraged students to make use of e-mail to communicate and the World Wide Web to help compensate for reduced in-person access to libraries. To test for such an effect, the authors queried graduates about their use of various technologies, both while still a student and later, after graduation. Graduates were asked whether they regularly used e-mail, and whether they used the World Wide Web to get information. In addition, they were asked whether they had participated after graduating in at least one ITV training or workshop or staffing. Each item was checked yes or no. The means for the items are shown for the three categories of graduates in Tables 6 and 7. The closer to 1 (yes) the scores were, the higher the proportion of graduates in that category who used the technology.

Contrary to expectations, the traditional graduates appear to have made *more* use of e-mail and the Web than did the full-ITV graduates. It is possible that this difference is due in part to reduced access of the full-ITV respondents to computer labs while in the MSW program. As noted earlier, full-ITV graduates rated access to resources such as computer labs lower than did traditional graduates. Unfortunately, the question on access to resources does not break down the responses to specific types of resources.

Traditional graduates varied in comparison with partial-ITV graduates on use of these technologies.

TABLE 6. Use of Technology While in the MSW Program

Items*	Full-ITV (n = 15)	Partial-ITV (n = 27)	Traditional (n = 25)	Grand means (n = 67)
Used WWW	1.47 (0.52)	1.33 (0.48)	1.24 (0.44)	1.33 (0.47)
Used e-mail	1.67 (0.49)	1.41 (0.50)	1.20 (0.41)	1.39 (0.49)

* Possible ratings were 1 = yes, 2 = no.
( ) = S. D.

TABLE 7. Use of Technology After Graduation

Items*	Full-ITV (n =15)	Partial-ITV (n = 27)	Traditional (n = 25)	Grand means (n = 67)
Used WWW	1.47 (0.52)	1.15 (0.36)	1.28 (0.46)	1.27 (0.45)
Used e-mail	1.47 (0.52)	1.22 (0.42)	1.24 (0.44)	1.28 (0.45)
Participated in at least one ITV training/workshop/staffing	1.67 (0.49)	1.74 (0.45)	2.00 (0.00)	1.82 (0.38)

* Possible ratings were 1 = yes, 2 = no.
( ) = S.D.

The only technology used more (after graduation) by full-ITV graduates was participation in an ITV training, workshop, or staffing. Both full-ITV (mean = 1.67) and partial-ITV (mean = 1.74) graduates had some experience with ITV training/workshop/staffing, while no traditional graduates (mean = 2.00) had this kind of ITV experience. The "spillover," if any, seems limited to ITV itself, but it could also be that ITV meetings are now in greater use in rural areas, where most full-ITV graduates work and where travel costs are greater, than in the Twin Cities, where most of the traditional graduates work.

When technology usage is compared before and after graduation within each category, it appears that full-ITV graduates' mean usage of e-mail increased, but not the mean usage of the Web. Partial-ITV graduates' mean usage increased a small amount for both media, while traditional graduates' mean usage decreased a small amount for both media.

DISCUSSION AND IMPLICATIONS FOR SOCIAL WORK EDUCATION

ITV and Program Support. Little difference was found between full-ITV and traditional graduates in their perceptions of their connections to the school and in their relationships with instructors. This finding is reassuring, since many faculty members and administrators are concerned that distance students may feel very isolated from the sponsoring institution (Coe & Elliot, 1997). Moreover, full-ITV graduates' rating of staff support for students was considerably *higher* than traditional graduates' perceptions. This higher rating is probably a result of the School's substantial investment in staff support for distance students, including assignment of a MSW-level coordinator to classes at each distant site, substantial training and supervision of these site coordinators, assignment of teaching assistants to each distance course at the originating site, a required visit to the remote sites by the instructors, and site coordinator and instructor availability before and after class. This investment may also account for full-ITV graduates' higher rating for access to relevant course materials, in comparison to traditional graduates. These findings confirm the importance of investing in supports for distance students, even though it adds considerably to program cost. There is a growing realization that distance education programs do not save money compared to traditional programs. However, they do enable institutions to reach student audiences that hitherto found graduate education inaccessible. This is an important consideration for all institutions of higher education, but especially so for land grant institutions like the University of Minnesota.

The two aspects of program support which received lower ratings from full-ITV graduates than from traditional graduates were students' connections to other students and adequacy of access to resources (e.g., library, copying, computer labs). Neither of these findings is surprising. It is understandably more difficult for students at one location to relate to students at another location, because there is no opportunity for before- and after-class socialization and the televised image of students at another location is quite small, even when the camera has zoomed in on the student speaker. Paradoxically, however, the students at a particular remote site sometimes build even stronger relationships with other students at that site than typically occur in the traditional classroom setting (Macy, 1999). This is probably not due to the ITV technology itself, but instead is a result of students at the remote site taking so many of their classes together and thereby coming to know each other very well.

Instructors in the University of Minnesota distance MSW program utilize several techniques to help build community among students across sites. First, all students are brought together in the same physical location for one class session early in the course. Second, instructors are encouraged to try to stimulate cross-site dialogue between students at different sites. Exercises, including roleplays, are sometimes structured so that students at one site must interact with students at another site. However, these techniques in themselves apparently were not fully adequate to bridge the distance between sites. Perhaps this is an inherent attribute of distance education. However, there may be ways in which other technologies can help to reduce the gap. The MSW program studied began in 1999-2000 to offer Web-enhanced courses, using WebCT software. While this technology is expected to benefit both traditional and distance MSW students, it may have special utility for increasing cross-site communication among students. WebCT is designed to easily facilitate the use of course chat rooms, discussion groups, bulletin boards, and e-mail (Wernet & Olliges, 1998). These features may enable students to relate more to each other both within and across sites (Mills & Payne, 1998; Huff & Johnson, 1998).

WebCT may also help the program address the second issue: better access to resources. Part of the problem of accessing resources for these distance learners is that most ITV courses are offered on the weekends. Students driving in to the remote site sometimes find the campus libraries and computer labs on reduced hours or closed entirely. Software like WebCT enables instructors to post a wide variety of materials, including articles, as well as syllabi and lecture notes. Likewise, the University of Minnesota libraries initiated in fall 1999 an electronic reserve system for distance courses as part of its overall effort to make its libraries more accessible to remote users. (See their website for distance learning services at *www.lib.umn.edu/dist/*.)

As more and more students purchase computers on their own or gain access through their employment, the issue of access to computer labs on weekends at distant sites may diminish. In the meantime efforts are underway to expand the weekend hours of libraries and computer labs at those sites.

ITV Impact on Use of Technology. The speculation that exposure to ITV might have a positive impact on adoption of electronic technologies such as e-mail and use of the World Wide Web was not supported by the data. There was, however, higher usage of ITV conferencing by both full-ITV and partial-ITV graduates than by traditional graduates. Some of this difference could possibly be due to the growing utilization of ITV for training of rural practitioners to save travel costs. However, the partial-ITV graduates, who tend to work more in urban than in rural areas, also reported higher post-graduate usage of ITV than did traditional graduates. The latter also tend to work in urban areas. Unfortunately the questionnaire did not ask whether the respondent's work location was urban or rural, so a more precise analysis of this data was not possible, but this question is planned for next year's survey.

ITV Impact on Learning. Full-ITV graduates generally were positive about their learning through the ITV-based MSW program. Over seventy percent indicated either that ITV delivery made no difference to their learning compared to traditional classroom courses or that ITV delivery actually enhanced their learning. Partial-ITV graduates were not quite as enthusiastic, however, with only half indicating that ITV either enhanced learning or made no difference to learning.

Possible explanations for the more favorable view by full-ITV graduates could be: (a) they simply had no other means than ITV for accessing the MSW degree and were therefore more appreciative of the opportunity, or (b) they had no concurrent non-ITV (traditional) courses for comparison, and therefore tended to rate them higher than did partial-ITV graduates, or (c) the numbers of respondents in each category are small and the difference is due simply to chance. Therefore the higher rating of ITV by the full-ITV graduates must be viewed cautiously. Yet, even if the rating of ITV MSW course delivery made by the partial-ITV graduates is the more valid rating (because those graduates had a better basis for comparison), the rating *at worst* suggests that ITV does almost as well as traditional classroom courses. If there is at the same time a big gain in opening access to MSW education for students living at considerable distance from schools of social work, one can argue that offering graduate social work education with only a small difference in learning effectiveness is indeed justified. While more research is needed comparing learning effectiveness for ITV and traditional MSW programs, there is growing evidence that the differences between the two formats are not great (Rooney et al., 1999; Hollister & McGee, 1998). It seems likely that distance education in social work will continue to grow in the years ahead.

This exploratory study has identified some areas for improvement in one ITV MSW program. The number of respondents, however, was small, and they were all graduates of one school of social work. Additional studies are needed of the questions raised here, both from analysis of additional data still to be collected from future cohorts of graduates of this same program, and from data from other ITV MSW programs.

REFERENCES

Coe, J. A., & Elliot, D. (1997, March). *An evaluation of teaching direct practice in distance education programs in rural settings*. Paper presented at the Annual Program Meeting of the Council on Social Work Education, Chicago, IL.

Hollister, C. D., & McGee, G. (1998). Delivering substance abuse and child welfare content through interactive television. *Proceedings of the Conference on Information Technologies for Social Work Education and Practice* (pp. 196-202). Columbia: University of South Carolina College of Social Work.

Huff, M., & Johnson, M. (1998). Students' use of e-mail and a listserv in distance education courses. *Proceedings of the Conference on Information Technologies for Social Work Education and Practice* (pp. 203-211). Columbia: University of South Carolina College of Social Work.

Kalke, N., Rooney, R., & Macy, J. (1998, March). *Providing effective education in distance education*. Paper presented at the Annual Program Meeting of the Council on Social Work Education, Orlando, FL.

Macy, J. A. (1999). *Exploring the experiences of social work graduate students who have completed their degrees via interactive television*. Unpublished doctoral dissertation, University of Minnesota.

Mills, R., & Payne, T. (1998, August). *Students using the web: Projects presented via WebCT.* Paper presented at the Conference on Information Technologies for Social Work Education and Practice, Charleston, SC.

Rooney, R., Freddolino, P., Hollister, C., & Macy, J. (1999, March). *Evaluating distance programs in social work: What does it all mean?* Paper presented at the Annual Program Meeting of the Council on Social Work Education, San Francisco, CA.

Wernet, S., & Olliges, R. (1998). The application of WebCT (Web Course Tools) in social work education. *Proceedings of the Conference on Information Technologies for Social Work Education and Practice* (pp. 304-310). Columbia: University of South Carolina College of Social Work.

Creating a TeleLearning Community for Training Social Work Practitioners Working with Troubled Youth and Their Families

Philip M. Ouellette
Scott Sells

SUMMARY. With the advent of several new communication technologies and the improvement of Web-based instructional software, combining several technology-supported teaching media may be a viable added dimension to consider when teaching advanced social work practice courses. What follows is a description of how faculty from two separate universities collaborated to create a dynamic telelearning community to train social work practitioners working with troubled youth and their families. By combining different technology-supported teaching media such as teleconferencing and a Web-based instructional environment, a unique "hi-tech" learning atmosphere evolved. Conditions that facilitate or hinder learning efficacy are explored as well as systemic challenges. *[Article copies available for a fee from The Haworth Document Delivery Service: 1-800-342-9678. E-mail address: <getinfo@haworthpressinc.com> Website: <http://www.HaworthPress.com> © 2001 by The Haworth Press, Inc. All rights reserved.]*

KEYWORDS. Distance education, web-based instruction, telelearning community, teleconferencing

Philip M. Ouellette is affiliated with the University of South Florida.
Scott Sells is affiliated with Savannah State University.

[Haworth co-indexing entry note]: "Creating a TeleLearning Community for Training Social Work Practitioners Working with Troubled Youth and Their Families." Ouellette, Philip M., and Scott Sells. Co-published simultaneously in *Journal of Technology in Human Services* (The Haworth Press, Inc.) Vol. 18, No. 1/2, 2001, pp. 101-116; and: *Using Technology in Human Services Education: Going the Distance* (ed: Goutham M. Menon, and Nancy K. Brown) The Haworth Press, Inc., 2001, pp. 101-116. Single or multiple copies of this article are available for a fee from The Haworth Document Delivery Service [1-800-342-9678, 9:00 a.m. - 5:00 p.m. (EST). E-mail address: getinfo@haworthpressinc.com].

As social work educators increasingly move toward integrating the use of new communication technologies and Web-based educational environments into existing classroom-designed courses, interesting shifts are being witnessed in how instruction is being delivered and how students learn. As a result, new learning environments are increasingly becoming available for social work students. Instruction is slowly moving from a mode of teacher-student interaction occurring in fixed locations at specified times to one in which students can access instructional resources from a variety of technology-supported learning environments regardless of one's location and at the student's convenience. This is becoming possible because several new technologies have matured to such an extent that instruction can be delivered to students on the campus, in their homes, or in their work places (Baker & Gloster, 1994).

This paper describes how social work educators from two different schools of social work pooled their resources and mutual expertise to co-teach an advanced family practice course for working with difficult children and adolescents entirely through the use of multiple technology-supported instructional environments. The teaching team used teleconferencing as an alternative to the classroom and a Web-based instructional environment to enhance the telelearning experience of weekly teleconference seminars. Tentative conclusions with respect to the strengths and weaknesses of each technology-supported instructional medium are outlined.

SHIFTING EDUCATIONAL PARADIGMS

The educational paradigm that has governed most of our colleges and universities to date is one that defined a college or university as an institution that exists to provide instruction (Barr & Tagg, 1995). Subtly but profoundly, the rapid growth of new information technology and advanced communication networks and its increase use within existing conventionally taught courses is forcing educators to re-examine not only the way instruction is delivered, but also question the very core of traditionally accepted pedagogical principles used to guide current teaching strategies. The gradual shift occurring in many educational settings is towards a paradigm that recognizes the educational institution as existing primarily to produce learning by whatever means necessary. As more emphasis is placed on the importance of learning outcomes, learning changes from a teacher-driven process where the instructor is the primary source of new information to an environment where the learner is increasingly empowered to direct his or her own learning process. In a student-centered learning paradigm, the role of the educator shifts from primary instructor to one of becoming more of a guide in the learning journey of students. Through ongoing peer interaction, students are empowered to take charge of their own learning as they discover knowledge for themselves, making learning a student-driven process.

TEACHING WITH TECHNOLOGY

Because of the development of several new instructional software programs now available to educators and the improvement of teleconferencing technology, instruction can be delivered to students on campus, in their homes, or in their work places (Baker & Gloster, 1994). The idea of implementing the "Virtual Classroom" as a viable added dimension to the learning process for human services practice courses has been explicated elsewhere (Ouellette, 1999). Essentially, a Virtual Classroom Pedagogical Strategy (VCPS) involves designing a series of Internet-based active learning activities (Misale et al., 1996; Hollings-worth et al., 1998) that provide students with the opportunity to not only acquire new information from a variety of sources, but to interact with peers and instructors about their evolving thought processes without the barriers of fixed locations and rigid time schedules. In addition to the Internet, teleconferencing technology permits the instructor to bring the classroom to the student at a distance.

The use of two-way video/two-way audio is the one technology-mediated instructional environment that most resembles the actual classroom setting. Although a number of resources have been made available to facilitate teaching in a teleconferencing environment (Cyris & Smith, 1990), the use of active learning strategies proposed by a number of educational experts to improve regular classroom teaching (Silberman, 1996; Bonwell & Eison, 1991) appears to enhance the learning performance of students when skillfully adapted to a technology-mediated environment. Designing a technology-mediated learning environment appears to be well suited for the educator that adheres to an educational paradigm where the student is considered the main agent in the process of discovery, not the teacher.

Research on the use of technology-mediated instruction has had a tendency to focus on comparing learning efficacy between classroom-based instruction and technology-supported environments (Beare, 1989; Haynes & Dillon, 1992; Hobbs, 1990). Not surprisingly, results have not been conclusive. Instead of comparing technology-supported instructional media to conventional classroom learning environments, the time has come to begin assessing which instructional medium is (i) best suited for what type of student, (ii) which best accomplishes what specific learning outcome, and (iii) which pedagogical principle is best operationalized by a particular medium. What follows is a description of how teleconferencing and a Web-based instructional environment were merged to create a dynamic learning experience in clinical social work for working with difficult children and their families.

THE TRAINING CONTEXT

Description of the Course: Treating children and adolescents with severe behavioral problems challenges even the most skilled social work practitioner. Practitioners typically have not received adequate preparation or training that provide step-by-step guidelines that facilitate working with this difficult and specialized population. Consequently, a course designed to meet the needs of practitioners working with this population was selected as the setting deemed most appropriate for implementing a technology-supported instructional strategy. The course is largely based on a model developed by the research work of Scott Sells (1998) where special youth problems are addressed by presenting a family-based model that articulates how to engage the uncooperative child or adolescent in the treatment process using age appropriate strategies.

The goal of the course was to provide a learning context where students could develop knowledge and skills in empowering parent(s), changing and shaping parent-child communication, and restoring nurture and tenderness to the child-parent relationship. The course provides students with a structure for intervening with families within multiple systems and as a part of a multi-disciplinary treatment team.

Teaching Strategies: A team-teaching instructional strategy was used within the technology-supported learning environment, irrespective of the medium used. This enabled two instructors at different sites to combine resources and expertise to create a context for learning.

The technology permitted the use of film of real cases to demonstrate intervention strategies as well as provide opportunities for students from all sites to actually participate in the observation of live therapeutic sessions in process. In addition to the resources available from the teaching team, students were provided an opportunity to see how theory and practice intersect by exposure to nationally known experts in the field of family therapy and play therapy. Combining didactic and experiential components to learning through Web-based assigned tasks and projects enabled students to integrate theory and practice.

The Training Sites: The two training sites and training groups chosen for this technology-mediated project were graduate classes associated with the Department of Social Work at Savannah State University, and the School of Social Work at the University of South Florida. Following the same course syllabus, course guide, and course evaluations, students from the both sites came together weekly for a three hour teleconference meeting with the teaching team. In addition to the teleconferencing medium, students were provided an opportunity to sign on an interactive course Web site developed and managed at the University of South Florida. The Web site provided a mechanism for students to download relevant course materials, acquire information on assigned tasks, read course notes and instructor slide presentations, as well as track individual performance. In addition to the access of online course information, the course Web site provided a means for students from all teleconferencing sites to post personal reflections on the class bulletin board, interact with one another through e-mail, and participate in synchronous exchanges through the class chat room.

Course Objectives: The course had eight specific learning objectives. After completion of the course, students would be able to:

- Conduct a comprehensive evaluation of difficult children within the context of environmental factors and developmental factors. Demonstrate an ability to understand the factors that cause and support behavioral problems in children and adolescents;
- Integrate the conceptual framework of family systems theory and other family intervention models (Structural, Strategic, Solution Focused, Life Model) into intervention strategies based on presenting problems and family dynamics;

- Integrate advanced practice skills into the formulation of a comprehensive case plan in families with difficult children and adolescents which are age appropriate;
- Apply specific principles and guidelines to engage uncooperative children, adolescents and adults; empower single parents and parents; change and shape parent-child communications; restore parental nurture and tenderness;
- Function effectively across multiple systems when working with difficult children and adolescents and their families (courts, school, work, other professionals);
- Evaluate the role of diversity in treatment and develop interventions which validate and support the rights and dignity of all family members;
- Examine the relevant research and technological advances within each treatment strategy to determine the relative strengths and weaknesses of various interventions with specific families;
- Learn and apply specific principles and guidelines on how to work with special treatment issues and populations, including: single-parent families, sexual abuse and trauma, abuse of alcohol and other drugs.

Evaluation and Feedback: For grading purposes students were required to complete three major learning activities. These activities included (1) participation in weekly Web-based learning assignments posted on the course Web site, (2) completion of a self-evaluation instrument regarding their telelearning experience, and (3) a personal reflection log collected for evaluation and feedback four times during the semester. To acquire data on student perception of their learning outcomes, a pre and post self-evaluation questionnaire was administered to students with respect to the course learning objectives. Students were to view and download the questionnaire from the course Web site and return the results to their respective instructors via the use of the class e-mail system. Table 1 is an example of one of the pre-test questionnaires.

Active Learning Strategies: A number of assignments were developed as learning strategies specifically designed for the electronic medium being used. For example, in the Web-based instructional environment, each on-line assignment included an element in which students were to interact either with one another or with the professors on some

TABLE 1

Working with Difficult Children and Adolescents:
Special Treatment Issues
Pre-Test

Rank your knowledge and skills on these 8 course objectives using the following Likert scale: 5 = completely competent and 1 = no knowledge or skills.

Course Objectives:
I am able to:

_____ 1. Conduct a comprehensive evaluation of difficult children within the context of environmental factors and developmental factors. Demonstrate an ability to understand the factors that cause and support behavioral problems in children and adolescents;

_____ 2. Integrate the conceptual framework of family systems theory and other family intervention models (Structural, Strategic, Solution Focused, Life Model) into intervention strategies based on presenting problems and family dynamics;

_____ 3. Integrate advanced practice skills into the formulation of a comprehensive case plan in families with difficult children and adolescents which are age appropriate;

_____ 4. Apply specific principles and guidelines to engage uncooperative children, adolescents and adults, empower single parents and parents, change and shape parent-child communications, restore parental nurture and tenderness;

_____ 5. Function effectively across multiple systems when working with difficult children and adolescents and their families (courts, school, work, other professionals);

_____ 6. Evaluate the role of diversity in treatment and develop interventions which validate and support the rights and dignity of all family members;

_____ 7. Examine the relevant research and technological advances within each treatment strategy to determine the relative strengths and weaknesses of various interventions with specific families;

_____ 8. Learn and apply specific principles and guidelines on how to work with special treatment issues and populations, including: single-parent families, sexual abuse and trauma, abuse of alcohol and other drugs.

Submit to the instructor via e-mail.

theme covered in the teleconferencing sessions. Tables 2 and 3 describe one example of an on-line learning assignment that was used to encourage peer and instructor interactions between course participants.

In the teleconferencing context the instructors used active learning strategies to engage student interaction in the different training sites. The strategy most often used was the probing question period. This involved posing questions to the students at several points during the instructors mini-lecture or presentation of a particular theme. Following active learning strategies suggested by Rosman (1985), the different types of questions an instructor might ask within a teleconferencing session may be categorized as in Table 4.

TABLE 2

On-Line Learning Assignment (Part I)
SOW xxxx Working with Difficult Children and Adolescents
Semester: Spring
Online Assignment: The Live Family Session – Week 7 (Part I)
Time: Estimated completion time: 1 hour
Time Frame to complete task: 2 weeks
Step #1: Recall the Live Interview conducted by Dr Sells in Session #7. Think of one or two "curve balls" the client-family directed at Dr Sells.
Step #2: Now before proceeding to the next step, think about how you might have responded or reacted to the client-family if you would have been confronted with these "curve balls." Write your thoughts on a piece of paper.
Step #3: Go to Dr Sells' Discussion Forum by clicking on the "bulletins" icon in the left frame.
Click on "Forum" in the menu. Select Dr Sells' Forum. Now click Instructor message #424, read the instructions, and post your responses or reactions.
Note: To post your responses or reactions, read the "Instructor message" on the bulletin board, click on "Quote" in the menu (on top), and type in your responses in the dialogue box.
Go to Part II Return to Assignment list. (Click "contents" above left)

TABLE 3

On-Line Learning Assignment (Part II)

SOW xxxx Working with Difficult Children and Adolescents

Semester: Spring

Online Assignment: The Live Family Session - Week 7 (Part II)

Time: Estimated completion time: 1 hour

Time Frame to complete task: 2 weeks

Step #1: Recall the Live Interview conducted by Dr Sells in Session #7. Think about similar "curve balls" client-families have directed at you in your internship experience. (Write one example on a piece of paper that illustrates this situation.)

Step #2: If you are an SSU student, go to Dr Ouellette's Discussion Forum. If you are a USF student, go to Dr Sell's Discussion Forum. (You may go directly to these forums by clicking on the "bulletins" icon in the left frame. Then, click on "Forum" in the menu. Select Dr Sells' Forum or Dr Ouellette's Forum.)

Step #3: Now click Instructor message #425 (Sells) or #426 (Ouellette), read the instructions, and post your example of a "similar curve ball" or dilemma. (Click on "Quote" in the top menu.)

Step #4: If you are a USF student, return to Dr Sells' Discussion Forum. If you are an SSU student, return to Dr Ouellette's Discussion Forum. (You may go directly to these forums by clicking on the "bulletins" icon in the left frame. Then, click on "Forum" in the menu. Select Dr Sells' Forum or Dr Ouellette's Forum.)

Step #5: Select a scenario posted by one of the students in the Discussion Forum. (Select one which no one else has selected or responded to. If they all have been responded to, select one at random.) Respond to or describe how you would react to your colleague's dilemma.

Note: To post your responses or reactions, read the "Instructor message" on the bulletin board, click on "Quote" in the menu (on top), and type in your responses in the dialogue box.

Return to Top of Page
Return to Assignment list. (Or click "contents" above left)

TABLE 4

Teleconferencing Sessions
Active Learning Strategies: The Probing Question Period
Questions that may be asked are: - Exploratory questions such as "What are the facts?"
- Challenge or testing questions such as "Are these solutions or interpretations adequate to the problem?"
- Contextual and relational questions such as "How is this solution like that solution? How is it different?"
- Priority questions such as "Which do you think is the best solution for the presented situation?"
- Concluding and conceptualizing questions such as "What have we learned from this interview?"

LESSONS LEARNED

Most students involved in this telelearning experience reported a positive learning experience. When combining several technological media to deliver instruction such as this experience exemplified, a number of lessons have been learned at multiple levels of the learning context, that is, at the student level, the instructor level and at the level of the organizational context.

At the Student Level: What was most evident at the student level was the need to adequately prepare students for the instructional medium being used. For most social work students, learning issues related to social work practice via a technological medium is an entirely new learning experience. Much student anxiety is expressed in various ways such as the exorbitant need to ask questions regarding course expectations, course requirements and course content. This suggests that instructors need to have sufficient preparatory time with students at each training site before coming on-line. Sufficient time must be devoted to properly prepare students for the teleconferencing environment, and a series of Web-based orientation exercises must be incorporated within the preparation phase of the course to assist students to learn how to navigate an interactive course Web site. This can do much to alleviate unnecessary use of on-line questions related to student fears, anxiety and technical difficulties.

Another factor to be aware of when combining several technologies for course instruction is the degree to which each an electronic medium requires a change in the student's traditional learning culture. For example, the teleconferencing environment appears the closest to an actual classroom setting. Like the traditional classroom, students come together at a specified time and at a designated place where teleconferencing facilities are available. And not unlike the classroom, the student listens attentively to the instructor(s) presentation, takes notes, and responds to questions when asked. Much of the learning process in a teleconferencing environment is teacher-driven. When students move to a Web-based instructional environment between teleconferencing sessions, the learning process shifts dramatically. The student must be sufficiently self-directed to explore the course Web site's content and learning activities at his own pace and at times convenient to his/her schedule. Most of the learning activities designed for the Web-based learning environment required some form of peer-to-peer or student-instructor interaction. Because most communication tools in a Web-based instructional environment tend to be a text-based mode of communication, students are required to think more about the nature of their responses. At first glance, a Web-based environment may appear to students as more intense and demanding more of their time. The nature of the environment requires a shift in what students are usually accustomed to with respect to the way one learns. That is, the student is required to move from a teacher-driven learning process in a teleconferencing environment to a student-driven learning process in a Web-based instructional environment. For some students, this may represent a major difficulty.

At the Instructor Level: One of the most important factors learned at the instructor level, especially when using a team-teaching instructional format, is to allow for sufficient pre-class preparation time for ongoing teacher conferences. The technology-supported instructional environment must mirror the teaching format that is being utilized. If a team teaching format is used between training sites, instructors must be equally present both in the teleconferencing environment and in the Web-based instructional environment. This ensures instructor team work and provides for modeling a true learning community in a telelearning environment.

In a teleconferencing context it has been found important for instructor presentations not to exceed 15 minutes without some opportunity for student input through some active learning strategy such as probing questions. Longer presentations have a tendency to make students at the remote sites feel isolated and unimportant. What has been found useful is to request students from one site to ask questions and require students from a different site to answer. This allows for exchanges between students at multiples sites. Although Power Point presentations and/or transparencies are useful visual media that complement a teleconference mini-lecture, it is important that long text be avoided and that images and text be clearly seen.

One of the most surprising results at the instructor level was the importance of ensuring that the instructor team equally support the use of all technological media being used for the delivery of a particular course. For example, one must avoid making Web-based assignments available for students in one training site but not the other. If all technology media are not used equally by all students in each training site, the tendency will be for students to only use the medium demanding the least effort. Making a Web-based learning environment optional and teleconferencing required provides a context for unequal participation in the overall telelearning experience. If multiple technology media are to be used, then it is important that all students experience the strengths that each medium provides.

Unanticipated was the amount of time that is required to design learning assignments and teaching strategies compatible to each technology-supported medium and the follow-up that is necessary to monitor student involvement. For example, Web-based learning assignments encouraged student interaction through the use of small group discussion forums. This requires active and persistent monitoring of student exchanges by the teaching team to ensure that discussion threads remain on topic. For team work to be effectively modeled, it was found important to ensure that all members of the teaching team be actively present in all the technology-supported teaching media that are used. Although it is time consuming, it is crucial to the modeling of team work and demonstrates effective collaboration among learners.

Another issue requiring time from instructors in a telelearning environment is student expectations for quick responses. Due to the easy access to professors via various communication tools, such as e-mail, chat rooms, and bulletin boards, students want and expect immediate feedback to dilemmas encountered. For example, after each Web-based learning assignment, students are able to provide immediate feedback to their instructors regarding the clarity of an assigned task. This requires instructors to constantly adjust their instructions to ensure clarity and expectations. Student input has suggested the importance for instructors to clearly define their instructions when providing an assigned task. Providing estimated time frames for completing tasks and the assignment of specific due dates has been found useful.

Although the question of preparation time is a concern expressed by many educators embarking on technology-supported teaching environments, it has not been considered taking much more preparation time than the time required of any collaborative "team teaching" effort used for a traditional classroom context. What has been found unique in a teaching environment using multiple technology-supported media is that collaborative efforts and team work among the instructor team must be consistent throughout the entire course delivery due to rapidity of the input and feedback received by students the technology-supported teaching mediums provide.

At the Organizational Level: The most surprising unanticipated outcomes of this project have been challenges experienced at the organizational and inter-organizational level. Although individual institutions may encourage their faculty to pursue distance education models of instructions, different academic departments have different financial resources and technical supports to realize such projects. At the institutional level, specific policies and procedures drive the use of certain technological facilities. Certain policies and procedures at publicly funded educational institutions can actually interfere with the effective implementation of technology-supported instructional environments and discourage team work and collaboration. For example, one institution may reserve the use of its teleconferencing facilities primarily for linking its own remote campuses. Others may prioritize in-state collaborative efforts. When a project such as the one implemented for this experience requires not only team work at the instructors' level but inter-organizational and inter-university collaboration, other more complex issues and questions arise. The following are a few of the questions collaborative teaching teams may wish to consider as they implement multiple technology-mediated learning environments such as teleconferencing and Web-based instruction:

- Does each training setting have similar teleconferencing hardware for a compatible teleconferencing connection?
- Are the technical supports sufficiently available at each training site to support faculty new to the use of this medium?
- How do students from different universities access a single university server for a course Web site if these resources are limited to students only enrolled at a specific university?
- When the educational program is made available to students at different universities and to students in different states, how is cost attributed? What is the cost of tuition? Who pays for what?
- Long distance connection fees can make technology-supported courses cost prohibitive for small institutions and groups in isolated communities. Who pays for telephone connection costs?

CONCLUSIONS

The experience of the authors in using multiple technology-mediated learning environments is forcing a re-examination of teacher roles. It appears that each technology-supported instructional medium has its own peculiar strengths and impacts teachers and students differently. In a traditional lecture-style instructional environment, whether it be classroom-based or teleconferencing, the teacher teaches, the teacher is the primary source of information, and the teacher is responsible for the quantity and quality of the teacher-student interactions which take place. Confirming what other educators have reported, with a Web-based instructional format, the teacher's role changes from that of instructor to facilitator (Berge, 1996). As one moves from a teleconferencing learning environment to a Web-based instructional environment the teacher becomes more of a guide for individual learners rather than a simple conduit for transmitting information. In addition, experience is showing that certain technology-supported learning environments, such as an Internet-based learning environment, enable students to discover knowledge for themselves especially when a series of action learning interactive activities are introduced. These activities also serve to enhance lecture-style instructional environments such as in-classroom or teleconferencing teaching environments.

By combining different technology-supported teaching strategies with a team teaching collaborative effort, it is becoming evident that the student's sole source of new information is no longer that of a single instructor but comes from a variety of sources. In addition, using multiple technological mediums to deliver course instruction has its own individual strengths and weaknesses. Along with its unique characteristics comes its unique challenges, as exemplified by the implementation of this project. When combining multiple technological teaching strategies it is important that we give serious consideration to facets unique at multiple levels of the learning context, that is, those challenges at the student level, the instructor level, and finally at the organizational or inter-organizational level.

The experience of this project is in line with evidence found by others in that learners learn best from opportunities to construct their own knowledge (Jonassen & Reeves, 1996; Kafai & Resnick, 1996). This suggests that there is no one set of pedagogical principles that fits all teaching media but rather, each technology-supported instructional format has its own unique strengths and pedagogical philosophy and each must be matched to specific learning objectives, individual learner styles, teacher flexibility, and organizational realities.

REFERENCES

Baker, W. & Gloster, A. (1994) Moving Towards the Virtual University: A Vision of Technology in Higher Education. *Cause/Effect, 17* (2), Summer.

Barr, R. & Tagg, J. (1995) "From Teaching to Learning: A New Paradigm for Undergraduate Education," *Change*, November/December 1995, 13.

Beare, P. (1989) The comparative effectiveness of videotape, audiotape, and telelecture in delivering continuing teacher education. *The American Journal of Distance Education. 3*(2): 57-66

Berge, Z.L. (1996). Changing roles in higher education: Reflecting on technology. *Collaborative Communications Review*. McLean, VA: International Teleconferencing Association. pp.: 43-53.

Bonwell, C. & Eison, J. (1991) *Active learning: Creating excitement in the classroom* (ASHE-ERIC Higher Education Report No. 1). Washington, DC: George Washington University.

Cyris, T.E. & Smith, F.A. (1990) *Telecourse teaching: A resource guide* (Second Ed.). Las Cruces, NM: New Mexico State University, Center for Educational Development.

Haynes, K. & Dillon, C. (1992) Distance education: Learning outcomes, interaction, and attitudes. *Journal of Education for Library and Information Science 33*(1): 35-45.

Hobbs, V. (1990) Distance learning in North Dakota: A cross-technology study of the schools, administrators, coordinators, instructors, and students. Two-way interactive television, audiographic tele-learning, and instruction by satellite. ERIC Document Reproduction Service ED 328 225.

Jonassen, D. H. & Reeves, T. C. (1996) Learning with technology: Using computers as cognitive tools. In D. H. Jonassen (Ed.) *Handbook of research for educational communications and technology.* New York: Macmillan. pp. 693-719.

Kafai, Y. & Resick, M. (Eds.) (1996) *Constructivism in practice: Designing, thinking, and learning in a digital world.* Mahwah, NJ: Lawrence Erlbaum.

Ouellette, P. (1999) Moving Toward Technology-Supported Instruction in Human Service Practice: The "Virtual Classroom." *Journal of Technology in Human Services, 16* (2/3) p. 97-111.

Rosmarin, A. (1985) The art of leading a discussion. In M. M. Gullette (Ed.) *On Teaching and Learning*. Cambridge, MA: Harvard-Danforth Center for Teaching and Learning. (pp. 34-39).

Sells, S. (1998) *Treating the Tough Adolescent: A Family-Based Step-by-Step Guide.* New York: Guildford Press.

Silberman, M. (1996) *Active learning: 101 strategies to teach any subject.* Boston: Allyn and Bacon.

e-Tools and Organization Transformation Techniques for Collaborative Case Management

Brenda Kunkel
Toni Yowell

SUMMARY. Welfare and workforce development reforms propel individual agencies into formal partnerships with one another. Collaborative Case Management is the cooperative delivery of social services to common clients. This paper describes technological tools and organization transformation issues for collaborative case management. A road map for a successful transition includes a shared vision, business/technology requirements, an information management strategy, redesigned jobs and processes, and a change management strategy. *[Article copies available for a fee from The Haworth Document Delivery Service: 1-800-342-9678. E-mail address: <getinfo@haworthpressinc.com> Website: <http://www.HaworthPress.com> © 2001 by The Haworth Press, Inc. All rights reserved.]*

KEYWORDS. Collaborative case management, technology transformation tools, technology transformation issues

RoseMarie is a social worker at the Tri-County One Stop Center. Her primary responsibility used to be case management for welfare clients, but her state recently restructured the agencies involved in delivering

---

Brenda Kunkel and Toni Yowell are affiliated with IBM.

[Haworth co-indexing entry note]: "*e*-Tools and Organization Transformation Techniques for Collaborative Case Management." Kunkel, Brenda, and Toni Yowell. Co-published simultaneously in *Journal of Technology in Human Services* (The Haworth Press, Inc.) Vol. 18, No. 1/2, 2001, pp. 117-134; and: *Using Technology in Human Services Education: Going the Distance* (ed: Goutham M. Menon, and Nancy K. Brown) The Haworth Press, Inc., 2001, pp. 117-134. Single or multiple copies of this article are available for a fee from The Haworth Document Delivery Service [1-800-342-9678, 9:00 a.m. - 5:00 p.m. (EST). E-mail address: getinfo@haworthpressinc.com].

welfare, employment and training, and vocational rehabilitation services. These agencies agreed to work together to serve shared customers through both co-located and virtual single points of entry. While she still manages welfare cases, RoseMarie is now using a collaborative case management model for delivering services to her clients.

Collaborative case management is the cooperative delivery of social services to common clients. The major activities within case management are intake, eligibility screening, assessment, enrollment, service plan development, activity tracking, follow-up and reporting. Collaboration among social service delivery programs can range from sharing information to joint responsibility for achieving an outcome with a common client. Through the use of collaborative case management the social service delivery system for a state or locality can leverage staff, physical, and funding resources with the goal of attaining self-sufficiency, security, and good health for shared clients in a more efficient and effective manner.

Best practices within the social service delivery field, and social work in particular, have moved to a holistic view of clients, their families, and their communities. Social workers have long been trained to work with clients and communities to change detrimental patterns and circumstances. However, most social workers leave their training to work in one of many distinct types of social service agencies, such as welfare, employment and training, or mental health. Each agency receives funding from different sources and each source brings restrictions and specific obligations for what a social worker may do with a client. Recent state and federal welfare and workforce development reforms provide social workers with an opportunity to influence agency leaders to take a more collaborative approach to managing the clients for whom they are responsible.

Collaborative case management requires a fundamental shift from policy-based decision making to information-based decision making. In this new collaborative information system, front-line social workers transform data into knowledge that enhances customer service with outcomes focused on client self-sufficiency, safety, and health. An information-based collaborative case management system requires a significant organization transformation, involving policies, technology, processes and managing the change.

The format of this article is to provide the reader with a glimpse into a day in the life of a social worker serving clients using a collaborative case management model. After briefly describing what our future social worker, RoseMarie, is doing at a given point in time, we describe the enabling technology and the relevant organization transformation issues. The article concludes with a road map for moving to a collaborative case management model.

ELECTRONIC SCHEDULING AND WORKFLOW MANAGEMENT

At 8:00 a.m. RoseMarie begins her day by communicating with her electronic office assistant. The voice response unit informs RoseMarie that she has three client meetings and an administrative chat room session scheduled today. Her tickler file indicates that Mrs. Stevenson should have completed her office skills certification and the system recommends sending an e-mail to obtain a copy. Today is RoseMarie's day to assist in the Intake Unit. She checks the electronic wait list to begin her preparation for meeting the first client.

e-Tool Description. RoseMarie's organization chose to use electronic scheduling and workflow management tools to dramatically increase staff efficiency and consistency. These tools include individual calendars, ticklers, resource scheduling and wait lists.

Groupware tools with calendar functions enable RoseMarie to keep an electronic calendar that she can share with peers. She also carries an electronic portable organizer that she updates to and from her desk top or laptop computer. The collaborative partnership agencies (the partners) keep a calendar for each client that allows the client anytime, anywhere access. It also makes referrals and activity coordination easier for social workers.

RoseMarie uses ticklers, which are notes that she writes to herself or a colleague asking to be reminded of a specific event at a specific date or time. The collaborative case management system also generates reminders that are created when certain information is entered. For example, the system could create reminders at the critical time points for a Temporary Assistance for Needy Families (TANF) recipient so that he did not lose days waiting for something to be scheduled or results to be shared.

Resource scheduling allows RoseMarie to know whether an event has availability or a resource is in use. Without this tool, a social worker will go through many time-intensive steps to schedule a resource. With the tool, a social worker can schedule the resource with the client still present to confirm her availability. Alternatively, the client can schedule the resource, using a kiosk or other networked computer, and the social worker can receive notification that this was done. The client's plan can automatically be updated using more complex technology.

Resource scheduling can also be used by agencies to schedule appointments on each other's calendars. For example, a local substance abuse treatment center may agree to allow the local One Stop Center to schedule substance abuse assessments on Tuesdays and Thursdays between 1:00 and 3:00 p.m. Both agencies can then view the availability of slots on a given day and plan accordingly.

Automated wait lists allow clients to register themselves for either a specific type of service or with a specific person or type of service provider. Flexibility built into the wait list tool could allow for daily changing of the wait list options so that sporadic events could have their own wait list on the days they occurred, for example interviews done by large employers once a month. A social worker could then select a client from the wait list and the appropriate form or action could be initiated.

RoseMarie saves time and hassles by using her electronic calendar, resource scheduler, tickler, and wait list. *Electronic scheduling and workflow management tools allow more effective use of time and reduce delays, oversights, and inconvenience.*

Organization Transformation. The collaborative partnership agencies, of which RoseMarie is an employee, are meeting the organizational challenges created by new legislation, budget constraints and changing client needs. The federal and state welfare and workforce development reforms changed the way the agencies operate, cooperate, and deliver services to clients. The "work first" approach and One Stop service delivery model established a renewed emphasis on collaborating to assist clients in attaining self-sufficiency.

The partners responded to the new requirements by breaking down stove-piped organizations and integrating processes and service delivery mechanisms. As the walls come down, organization strategies, budgets, and cultures collide. Agency identity and "turf" are at stake and the organizations must negotiate through a myriad of systems, policies and procedures that exist to meet specific goals.

Leaders cast aside "how business has always been done" and adopt a new, integrated vision. The common vision drives development of business requirements, again, all focused on client service delivery. Given the complex issues inherent in partnering, the leaders realized that it would take time to reach consensus on, develop, and implement new processes, standards and basic operating procedures. A phased approach would allow some flexibility and provide the time necessary to create additional buy in. They acknowledged that this was not necessarily the most efficient or cost-effective approach, but it was the most realistic. As a result the partners started the transition by defining common ground rather than letting differences stall the integration process. However, the differences are being addressed and resolved. *Leaders established a vision, mission, and strategy for combining services and major technology investments must support that strategy.*

As shown in the following diagram (see Figure 1), the partners moved from stove-piped processes to collaborative, integrated processes.

Process and job redesign decreases administrative time and frees up RoseMarie and her peers to use more advanced judgment and training-based skills. The organizational and technological changes open informa-

FIGURE 1

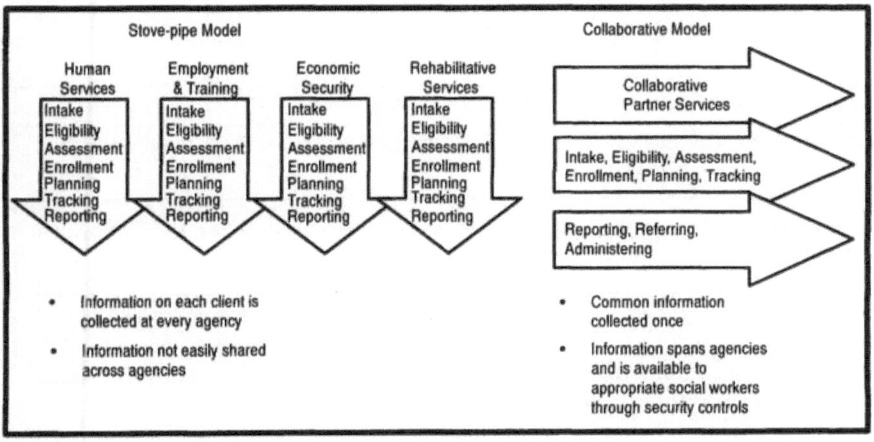

tion channels, automate repetitive information capture and procedures, and empower employees with the ability to cross over traditional organizational boundaries in serving a client. *The collaborative partnership agencies align redesigned jobs, processes, and technology with business requirements.*

When the partners made significant changes to their processes, structure, and technology they realized performance measures needed to change. The current trend in social services moves away from measuring outputs and moves toward measuring outcomes. Federal funding was previously tied to measures such as number of slots filled, number of clients served, and total program cost. Recent state and federal reforms shifted performance measurement to outcomes and enabled social workers to serve the total needs of their clients in an effort to achieve higher order outcomes of self-sufficiency, safety, and health. This shift allows the partners to apply resources in areas that derive the best outcomes. Table 1 contains typical outcome measures; this example is from the Welfare-to-Work program.

INTAKE AND ELIGIBILITY SCREENING

At 10:00 a.m. RoseMarie prepares to see a client new to the Tri-County One Stop Center. She uses the system to guide her through intake and eligibility screening.

RoseMarie goes to the Reception Area and calls her first client. Pat needs assistance in writing a resume and has a visual impairment.

TABLE 1. Typical Outcome Measures

Value/Outcome	**Performance Measure***
Placement in unsubsidized jobs	Number of clients employed in the target population
Duration of job placement in unsubsidized jobs	Number of placements in unsubsidized employment --- 6 months --- 12 months
Increase in earnings by individuals placed in unsubsidized jobs	Average earning of individuals at 6 months who obtain employment in unsubsidized jobs

*The partners define desired outcomes and corresponding performance measures.

RoseMarie sets Pat up in the resource room, which is designed for self-directed assistance. Pat will use the system to create a resume, schedule a role-play interview, and identify other programs for eligibility screening.

Prior to calling her next client on the Human Services waiting list, RoseMarie conducts an electronic search to determine if Chris received assistance from another state agency. Chris currently receives Unemployment Insurance, so the system populates all of the necessary forms with the information from the UI database. They discuss Chris's needs and then RoseMarie screens Chris for eligibility for services offered by all agency partners in the One Stop System.

e-Tool Description. Rose Marie was able to set Pat up in the Resource Room because the partners chose to use technology that gives clients more control over their use of the social service delivery system by allowing them to play a direct role in the service delivery process. When Pat decides to find out what else she may be eligible for, the computer asks her a series of questions. The partners chose a screening application that uses the answer from one question to determine which question to ask next. This makes the screening process faster and less confusing for Pat. When the electronic interview is complete, Pat receives a list of programs for which she may be eligible and she can choose to see why she was not eligible for other programs.

The eligibility-screening tool is part of the self-registration component of the partner's case management information system. Clients see information about the services offered by all partners, do a preliminary eligibility screening, select from local service providers offering the services for which they may be eligible, and, for some programs, begin to fill out the application. The application allows Pat to browse anonymously and to link to electronic services offered by any of the partners. *Interactive, intelligent tools give clients a stronger role in obtaining services.*

The partners not only needed to negotiate on the electronic tool they could all use for eligibility screening, but they also had to agree on how client information would get into and out of that application. Some of the collaborative partners could not afford a large technology investment while others were not dissatisfied with their current data gathering, storing and reporting capabilities. Therefore, the solution for communicating and collaborating with partners needed to leverage existing technology as much as possible. This requirement involved finding a way to share information between the different databases and applications, or legacy systems, of each of the collaborative partners.

Most of the collaborative partners chose to use the same application to gather the information they wanted to share. The partner that did not want to use a new application still shares intake information with the other partners. The shareable information gets translated into the software language spoken by the legacy systems of each partner. The collaborative information system is designed so that information is both taken from the legacy system to be used by the common application and taken from the common application to be used by the legacy system. The advantage to integrating legacy data into a common application is that during intake, RoseMarie could type in Chris's name, ask the system to search all of the partners' legacy systems for information on Chris, and then have the form she was using automatically filled in with that information.

The partners validated that the intake and eligibility screening tools met important business requirements:

- Focus on mission critical services. The collaborative case management information system made the partners more aware of what each has to offer a client. Partners now refer clients when their agency cannot meet a need rather than creating a new program. This benefit has been realized most significantly for support services like child care and transportation.
- Tailor service delivery to meet the unique needs of each client and give them a choice in how those needs may be met. The partnership maintains a database of all of the local service delivery providers. An electronic tool allows client needs to be matched against service provider characteristics.

An easily-accessible screening tool increased referrals between agencies because staff became cross-informed of each others' programs. The partners also found that clients spent less time in the service delivery system and were more satisfied because most of their needs were met with the right array of services through their first contact with the service delivery system.

The partners decided that the benefits of the common intake and eligibility screening components of the case management tool justified, and even demanded, that these components be web-enabled.

They believe that web-enabled self-registration will save staff time and enhance customer satisfaction. The partners envision the self-registration module available on the Internet, in their local offices, and even in kiosks in libraries or shopping malls. *Collaboration requires a strategy for sharing information among existing information systems.*

Organization Transformation. The technology vision of the partners moves them into the internet space to provide clients with increased access to services. They view this move as an evolutionary process rather than a revolutionary transformation. Currently, the agencies are at different points in terms of their Internet capabilities and philosophies.

Most partners *publish* information about programs and services. In addition, the web sites provide telephone numbers, local office locations, and operating hours. Partner agencies originally hesitated to move past publishing because of the perception that the clients most likely to use their services had no access to an electronic delivery system. Three factors pushed the partners beyond publishing. First, their shared vision includes minimizing the gap between the "computer rich" and poor. Second, the partners face continued budget pressures and the need to integrate service delivery, both of which electronic business assists in addressing. Third, clients already receive services from commercial entities through the Internet and they expect the same from government.

Several agencies moved into *informational* use of the Internet. In these agencies detailed information on services and government processes is available to clients. In addition, clients can download tools, such as forms. They no longer need to call or make a trip down to the local office. This decreased the need for some administrative staff coverage. Clients also e-mail social workers with specific questions, rather than go through telephone/voice mail channels. Service levels increased and social worker time on administrative tasks decreased.

The partners envision moving toward *transactional* and then *transformational* uses of the internet. Transactional uses would include real time interaction with government. Eligibility screening and scheduling for assessments could be accomplished "live" on-line, with intelligent systems prompting clients and providing information based on client answers. Transactional uses require limited integration of departments and this seems realistic based on the partners vision and planning strategy. Transformational uses would provide real-time query capability for employees and clients. The Internet would become integrated into the overall collaborative case management system. In addition to the self-registration module described above, the partners believe that the Internet can change the service delivery system in many ways, including:

- Contracted service providers could enter time and attendance, case notes, or other client specific information onto an electronic form that is then read by the collaborative case management information system which puts the information both in all of the forms required across the partner agencies for that particular client and in the integrated service plan
- Clients can schedule appointments over the Internet, be informed of the required documentation, scan that documentation into the system from wherever they are, and receive confirmation of their appointment and file status. This interaction is then logged into the related service plan(s).

The partners moved from a business vision of collaborative case management to defining business requirements to creating technology requirements. They built an Information Technology Strategic Plan to capture these requirements and assist them in deciding what their Internet strategy should be, what software they required, and what changes needed to be made to their technology infrastructure to allow them to achieve their vision. *The Internet is transforming the way the partners deliver social services.*

SERVICE DELIVERY PLANS

After lunch with nearby colleagues, RoseMarie conducts a home visit to update an existing client's Individual Service Plan. She uses her laptop computer and a state-of-the-art case management application that uploads to her electronic office assistant.

RoseMarie reviews Stacey Miller's service plan for employment and training. Her laptop provides RoseMarie with Stacey's previous plan as well as updated financial tracking information and target goals with intermediate steps. RoseMarie compares the plan against the trend information stored on her laptop. Together, RoseMarie and Stacey update Stacey's progress and revise activities and goals.

RoseMarie reviews, with Stacey, service plans for each of the children. They talk with Joey about his probation status. They schedule an assessment for Timmy's possible learning disability. Finally, they check on Kerry's Medicaid payment claim.

When RoseMarie arrives back at the office, she types in a case note for the family and replicates to the electronic office assistant.

e-Tool Description. The partners chose a collaborative case management application that allows RoseMarie to work while connected to the network at her office, while connected over the Internet from home or a partner's office, or while disconnected, such as from a client's home. The laptop that RoseMarie brings to the Miller's home contains all of the functionality of the application in her office, but only contains the files for her current caseload. Through replication, RoseMarie is able to download the most current version of the files that she needs and then later to upload her information into the common database. *Mobile computing give social workers greater flexibility in how and where they work.*

The collaborative information system gives each individual their own file, but also links that file to those with whom the individual has a relationship. In this way, each partner agency can create documents and track progress according to their requirements–either as an individual or as part of a grouping.

The assessment, enrollment, service plan development and activity tracking components of collaborative case management traditionally have been program specific. Until regulations change, each partner may have to maintain their own forms for these processes. However, the partners felt strongly that the benefit to the client was in creating an integrated service delivery plan. Therefore, their collaborative information system pulls from the plans maintained in the individual legacy systems and presents RoseMarie with an integrated plan. She can then make planning decisions based on the full continuum of services being provided to the Millers by all of the partners. The Tri-County One Stop Center took this one step further and made RoseMarie the primary case manager across all partners. As a result, she takes responsibility for connecting the Millers to the right person within each program, for monitoring progress across all service plans, and for convening cross-program strategy sessions to facilitate the delivery of the best array of services to meet the Millers' needs. The system notifies RoseMarie of significant status changes in any of the programs in which the Millers are involved.

Organization Transformation. When RoseMarie was given the capability of viewing information across agency lines, she was both encouraged and concerned. The increased accessibility to information allows a holistic approach to providing services to a family. However, she had reservations about sharing potentially confidential client information. She also was not certain that she could adequately guide clients through services that were not offered by her agency.

The partner agencies found that existing policies were preventing needed changes in business processes and technology that aimed at enhanced customer service. For example, organizations were often reluctant to unleash the full power of technology-enabled information sharing due to policies related to confidentiality. Conventional thinking advised that compartmentalization of information better protected client rights, and also maintained some measure of security. In addition, the social work ethical code advised against disclosing client information.

Today confidentiality is as important as ever, however, the information paradigm is shifting. Organizations expanded their definition of "need to know" and "can know" information related to clients. These agreed-upon definitions and procedures increased comfort that program-specific details about a client will not be disclosed. RoseMarie's agency provided rationale, processes and education on security issues to address confidentiality and privacy concerns. The partnership agencies continue to focus on issues related to vulnerability and risk for systems and data. They formed a cross-organization security team to identify and make recommendations pertaining to the issues. The team was comprised of social workers, information technology employees, policy makers, and legal advisors. The group defined six key security points:

- Integrity–protection against unauthorized modification or destruction of critical data;
- Access Control–security services to enforce the rights and privileges of authorized users;
- Availability–measures to prevent viruses or other code from disrupting the system;

- Authentication–ways to make sure that the user was correctly identified
- Non-repudiation–methods to provide proof of the origin and delivery of a message or data
- Confidentiality–protection against unauthorized disclosure of information or invasion of privacy.

The team recommended a comprehensive security policy. *Addressing real and perceived security issues builds confidence in the technology.*

ELECTRONIC TEAMWORK AND REPORTING

At 3:00 p.m. RoseMarie dials into an inter-agency chat session on a proposed policy to provide home computer terminals to families receiving state assistance. After the session, she verifies that electronic summary reports are sent to the main office.

Prior to the chat session, RoseMarie compiled statistics, via the internet, on poverty and the computer age. During the chat, she transmitted this information in a side-bar conversation to colleagues downstate. RoseMarie received an e-mail with a URL for a distance learning opportunity for using technology in group supervision. She "clicked" on the URL to download the course description.

At the end of the day, RoseMarie submitted a query on how many of the Center's families attending the local elementary school received Food Stamps. She intends to use the information to advocate for a greater share of state funds for her jurisdiction.

e-Tool Description. RoseMarie can participate in decision-making meetings that would be deemed "too much effort" if she needed to be physically present. As a result, front-line insight and information can influence policy setting.

As the partners move toward transformational use of the Internet in service delivery, RoseMarie and her peers will have access to a wider range of tools for finding, organizing, and sharing information. Currently, RoseMarie uses the collaborative information system to do ad hoc queries and reporting. The leaders in this partnership use the collaborative information system to comply with their individual reporting requirements.

The partners developed a common intranet, where knowledge is shared between employees and other organizations. In the past, agencies duplicated efforts and recreated similar types of information (best practices, policy interpretations). Also, contract service provider research was not readily available to all employees that could make productive use of the data. The agencies did not always have all the information they needed, or they had the information but could not locate it. In response to these difficulties and the paper intensive environment, the partners implemented a knowledge management system. They also use data mining capability for daily operational decisions and long-term planning. The decision support system used by the partners enables them to measure their progress toward their original vision. *Knowledge management turns data into information that can be used and shared.*

Organization Transformation. Collaborative case management involves significant changes for agencies and individuals. Unfortunately, employees often fear process redesign and technology insertion. They are not resisting change, but rather the way that it disrupts their lives. Major technology changes may result in:

- a perceived threat to job security,
- a shift in influence, authority and control,
- loss of expertise,
- a requirement to learn new skills,
- and, a change in the way it was always done before.

In order to counteract these fears, the partners developed and implemented an aggressive change management strategy, including a communication plan and a training plan. The change management strategy positioned them to deal with human reactions to organizational restructuring and new technology. It involved visible and committed leaders providing clear direction and articulating a compelling need for change. To effectively manage significant change, the partners helped employees understand the reasons for the change, created commitment to the new model, provided capabilities to make needed adjustments and tracked the process of change to make sure that it was happening. Even when employees understood the compelling reasons for change, they needed personal involvement to fully accept the changes. Types of involvement included opportunities to express concerns and input into new designs.

As a social worker, RoseMarie feels she is in a win-win situation.

She has opportunity to enhance her own job skills through exposure to a myriad of state programs that used to be stove piped by agency. In addition, she is on the cutting edge of technology. Not only are the technology skills marketable, but also the valuable time and resources she saves by using technology can be redirected toward serving her client.

The partners developed a comprehensive change management plan and involved social workers in determining products, services and system features.

Communication, or lack thereof, often sub-optimized the integration process. Early on, leaders recognized that good communication builds agency coalitions and peer relationships that support the new integrated model. However, reluctance to release preliminary plans and failure to solicit input moved the negative rumor grapevine into high gear. The partners finally developed a communication plan to address these problems. Key elements of their communication plan included downward flow, upward flow and horizontal flow of information related to the organization transformation. The partners found that in order for a person to truly receive a communication and accept its message, that person must understand it, believe that it reflects organizational goals and feel that it supports their interests. Also, the communication must be delivered in a timely manner. Effective upward communications from employees to managers and leaders required management involvement, active listening and action on ideas. Since the grapevine will always exist, leaders continue striving to create positive message traffic. *A comprehensive, proactive communication plan is essential.*

The Training Team, comprised of training professionals, technology specialists and users from multiple agencies, recommended a strategy to improve the social worker's ability to successfully use technology. The team developed a training philosophy to minimize time away from clients, while providing a phased approach to educating users on relevant topics. Computer-based training allowed social workers to improve their skills with new technology at their own pace. Classes provided over the internet allowed social workers to interact with their peers while remaining in their offices. Ever-increasing types of distance learning tools and strategies continue to simplify the effort required for social workers to increase their skills. In person training classes were also provided on an as needed basis. In addition, application training resident on the collaborative case management system included both help for how to use certain features and functions, as well as help specific to what the social worker is trying to do in a certain field in the application.

The partners built a support system that social workers can call regarding problems connecting to the network or performing a required procedure using the new technology. The support system has three key elements: peer support, process and procedure support, and the traditional technology help desk. The training team built an evaluation process and collected data on the value and impact of different types of training and support. *The partners developed training and support programs to ensure effective use of technology.*

ROADMAP TO COLLABORATIVE CASE MANAGEMENT

The transformation to a collaborative case management system requires a comprehensive approach to addressing business and technology requirements. In most social service agencies, business requirements are driven by legislative policy decisions. Information technology planning and implementation are based on business strategy and requirements. Table 2 summarizes key considerations for organization transformation and technology initiatives.

The road map described above applies to agencies wanting to use all of the tools and techniques described in this paper, as well as to those agencies attempting only a portion. Successful projects allow adequate time for a planning and assessment phase because rework costs far more, in terms of dollars and momentum, than building from consensus and strategy. The technology and business transformation components are interdependent. To implement only one will result in lost opportunity at best, and possibly in failure of the initiative. At the same time, people need to see action and celebrate success if they are to sustain their commitment to a new collaborative case management model. Therefore, leadership requires long term vision with a series of success points.

We are familiar with the efforts of several states to move to a collaborative case management model for social services delivery. The technology used or planned for in these initiatives varies widely. Most partnerships want to use an electronic government approach, however, they need to leverage their current technology investment. Therefore,

TABLE 2. Key Considerations for Organization Transformation and Technology Initiatives

Business Transformation	Technology Initiatives
Leaders established a vision, mission, and strategy for combining services and major technology investments must support that strategy.	
• The collaborative partnership agencies align redesigned jobs, processes, and technology with business requirements.	• Electronic scheduling and workflow management tools allow more effective use of time and reduce delays, oversights, and inconvenience.
• The partners define desired outcomes and corresponding performance measures.	• Interactive, intelligent tools give clients a stronger role in obtaining services.
• The Internet is transforming the way the partners deliver social services.	• Collaboration requires a strategy for sharing information among existing information systems.
• Addressing real and perceived security issues builds confidence in the technology.	• Mobile computing gives social workers greater flexibility in how and where they work.
• The partners developed a comprehensive change management plan and involved social workers in determining products, services and system features.	• Knowledge management turns data into information that can be used and shared.
• A comprehensive, proactive communication plan is essential.	
• The partners developed training and support programs to ensure effective use of technology.	

collaborative case management technology investments need to maximize use of current technology while enabling increased use of the Internet.

Compliance with the Workforce Investment Act has been the strongest motivator for adopting a collaborative case management model. States faced a July 1, 2000 deadline for implementing their One Stop initiatives. However, we also find that some states, counties, and localities have been using a collaborative case management model for quite a while. These efforts have often been informal and face tremendous policy barriers. The lessons learned from these earlier attempts suggest that once social workers from different agencies begin to work with and rely on one another on a regular basis, many of the change management issues discussed in this paper become much less significant. For instance, many partnerships report that their clients are very willing to sign release of information waivers because they see a benefit to themselves. We also find that partners respect each other's service delivery approaches and often revise procedures based on experience with another program's better way of doing certain activities.

Collaborative Case Management is the cooperative delivery of social services to common clients. Electronic tools and organization transformation techniques support multi-agency partnerships in their efforts to integrate service delivery and to allow clients to enter the service delivery system anytime, anyplace.

AUTHORS' NOTE

The authors wish to acknowledge our colleagues at IBM whose experience and expertise, combined with our own, provided the vision and direction for this document. Readers wishing additional information on the *e*-government tools and organization transformation techniques that support collaborative case management can visit the following web sites or contact the Social Services Solution Consulting and Integration practice principal, Pat Condon, at *pcondon@us.ibm.com* (301) 320-2424.

http://ec.fed.gov/
http://www.software.ibm.com/commerce/
http://www.ieg.ibm.com

Using Geographic Information System (GIS) Technology to Integrate Research into the Field Practicum

Robert L. Watkins

SUMMARY. This article reports on efforts to answer some basic questions arising in the introduction of technology into the social work curriculum. It involves an on-going project to integrate research into field instruction by training students to use Geographic Information System technology to identify and meet information needs of their field placement agency. Background on the project is given, with discussion of three concerns that shaped it. An explanation of how GIS works and how it can be used in the human service agency is provided, along with an account of the project's outcome. Preliminary conclusions regarding future efforts are offered. *[Article copies available for a fee from The Haworth Document Delivery Service: 1-800-342-9678. E-mail address: <getinfo@haworthpressinc.com> Website: <http://www.HaworthPress.com> © 2001 by The Haworth Press, Inc. All rights reserved.]*

KEYWORDS. Social work education, information technology, geographic information systems

For more than a decade, the growing importance of computers has focused attention on the need for social work education to prepare students to utilize information technology (e.g., Cnaan, 1988; Nurius,

---

Robert L. Watkins is Associate Dean for Academic Administration and Information Tech, Tulane School of Social Work, Tulane University, New Orleans, LA 70118-5672 USA (E-mail: rwatkins@mailhost.tcs.tulane).

[Haworth co-indexing entry note]: "Using Geographic Information System (GIS) Technology to Integrate Research into the Field Practicum." Watkins, Robert L. Co-published simultaneously in *Journal of Technology in Human Services* (The Haworth Press, Inc.) Vol. 18, No. 1/2, 2001, pp. 135-154; and: *Using Technology in Human Services Education: Going the Distance* (ed: Goutham M. Menon, and Nancy K. Brown) The Haworth Press, Inc., 2001, pp. 135-154. Single or multiple copies of this article are available for a fee from The Haworth Document Delivery Service [1-800-342-9678, 9:00 a.m. - 5:00 p.m. (EST). E-mail address: getinfo@haworthpressinc.com].

Hooyman & Nicoll, 1988). A number of strategies for introducing technology into the curriculum (Hernandez & Leung, 1990; van Lieshout & Roosenboon, 1995) and typologies of needed areas of competence (LaMendola, 1987) have been offered, but efforts to integrate training into the social work curriculum have also encountered obstacles ranging from "*ambivalence, ambiguity, and alienation*" (Nurius & Nicoll, 1989, p. 65) to lack of resources and time (England, Rivers & Watkins, 1999). As a result, while there is general recognition of the importance of information technology and the need to integrate it into the curriculum, integration does not seem to be happening on a large scale (Finn & Lavitt, 1995).

The introduction of information technology into the social work curriculum necessitates numerous decisions. In addition to developing an over-all strategy, desired levels of competence, and a model for instruction, there are issues of access, inclusion, and the allocation of time and resources that must be resolved. This paper describes an effort to begin to address some of those issues. At this point, it is premature to judge whether the decisions made were correct, but some preliminary conclusions can be drawn and will be offered at the end of the paper.

One of the problems facing educators is limited experience in instructional models for the introduction of technology. As Audet and Abegg (1996) point out, there are competing beliefs among cognitive scientists as to how technical knowledge is acquired, which impacts how instruction is delivered. At one end is the traditional classroom or lab approach, at the other, self-directed learning. At this point, it is not clear what approach works best, though we do know that no one approach works for everyone. So how might we begin in developing a model?

A basic question that can do much to frame later decision-making is whether students are to be trained to use computer applications–or are they to be trained to apply them? That is to say, is the emphasis to be on teaching students to use computers–or on how they can be used? As Turkle (1997a) puts it, should the goal be to develop "*fluency with software,*" or should we "*think of computer literacy as the ability to use the computer as an information appliance*"*?* The former approach emphasizes the development of the skills necessary to use applications, which may then be used to accomplish practical ends, and is more characteristic of the classroom approach. The latter approach focuses on a practical goal and then develops the skills needed to accomplish it, and while it may be used in the classroom, it is more characteristic of self-directed learning. Or should the approach simply be "*premised on the ability to learn from doing and to do from learning*" (Turkle, 1997b)? How these questions are answered does much to shape later decisions.

To be sure, a certain level of technical proficiency is necessary to utilize computers. One must know the mechanics of how hardware and software work to use the technology. But is this the kind of training that should become a part of the formal curriculum? Or should the expectation be that students will acquire a basic level of proficiency on their own? If so, how will issues of access and inclusion be handled in those cases where proficiency is lacking? Given the complexity of many applications, at what level is the standard of competency to be established? The need for answers to these questions underlies this project.

BACKGROUND ON THE PROJECT

This project was shaped by three concerns. First was recognition of the need to integrate information technology into the curriculum. Second was the perception among faculty teaching in the research and field sequences at Tulane that more integration of effort was necessary. And third was the belief of the author that social work needs to be more proactive in the use of information communication technologies. The search for a way to integrate these concerns led to this project.

Introduce Information Technology into the Social Work Curriculum

There was a general recognition by the faculty that information technology is a competency that social work students need to be equipped with. However, there was no accepted institutional approach to introducing it into the curriculum. While a required data analysis course involved the use of computers, the focus was on the use of data analysis software. The university library offered short courses in the use of the Internet for research, which students were encouraged to take, but no other formal programs were available. Given the time constraints of a crowded curriculum, a separate course to teach about computers was not feasible. How could the subject be introduced?

Increase Integration of the Curriculum

At Tulane, students are required to take a two semester, classroom-based research course. In the remaining two semesters, they conduct an independent research project, usually in groups. Students have full responsibility for designing and conducting the project, though they have the assistance of faculty research advisors. In a few cases, field placement agencies had research agendas, which they required students placed with them to work on. There was no formal coordination between the research and field sequences regarding agency-based research.

Prompted by problems some students were having at such a placement, the research sequence initiated a meeting with field coordinators to discuss what might be done to insure that students had a productive research experience. In the course of that meeting, it became clear that there were opportunities for students to conduct research projects meeting the real information need of placement agencies. However, it was not clear how to use these opportunities.

Introduce Technology into the Social Work/Human Service Community

It is generally accepted that human services are under pressure to do more with less. The shift in responsibilities from the federal to the state and local levels, as well as changing funding levels for human services, have spurred efforts to improve efficiency and effectiveness. One response has been computerization, particularly in what is now called "behavioral healthcare" (cf., Trabin, Ed, 1996.) However, the form this computerization has taken has prompted concerns about "rationalization" and the threat it poses to social work values (Phillips & Berman, 1995, pp. 10-26). The concern that developed is how to find ways whereby "*. . . harmonization between IT* [information technology] *and social work values can be maximized*" (Phillips & Berman, p. 135).

Genesis of the Project

With these three concerns, the question became how to leverage the effort to integrate technology into the curriculum and train students to use it, with the need to help agencies develop applications that met their needs. No one approach can meet all situations, but Wier and Robertson's (1998) article on "Teaching Geographic Information Systems in Social Work Education" suggested a possible vehicle. It prompted Internet research, which provided enough insight into potential applications to confirm the conclusion of Hoefer, Hoefer, and Tobias (1994) that it would be possible to use GIS technology *"to link social work practice, research, and education."*

WHAT IS GIS?

Geographic information system (GIS) technology is a computer-based tool for mapping and analyzing things that exist and events that happen on earth. (See Appendix A for a discussion of how GIS technology works, criteria for selecting software, and comparison of products evaluated for this project). GIS integrates common database operations that deal with data with the unique visualization and geographic analysis benefits offered by maps. These abilities distinguish GIS from other information systems and make it useful for explaining events, predicting outcomes, and planning strategies.

GIS facilitates the multiple level, visual display of data on a geographic background. Any quantitative or qualitative information that can be linked to a geographic reference point (e.g., street address or neighborhood boundary) can be depicted on a map. Depending on the purpose and nature of the data, it can be displayed in the form of points of different sizes, patterns of different colors and shading, and a variety of graphic symbols. Its power comes from the ability of the mind to distinguish pattern and color, making it possible to analyze, compare, and contrast vast quantities of quantitative data. Maps make it possible to see patterns and trends that would be difficult to detect looking at numeric data alone.

What Can Be Done with GIS?

The potential applications in human services are limited at this point only by our lack of experience and imagination. In the area of community building, the Department of Housing and Urban Development (1997) identified four main application areas:

1. Planning and implementing specific community initiatives
2. Assessing conditions and trends
3. Comprehensive strategic planning
4. Partnering in citywide initiatives and policy change.

Queralt and Witte (1998) described fifteen potential applications for practice, administration, and research:

- Inventory services provided and the clientele receiving them
- Document socio-demographic characteristics of the service area
- Forecast future needs of current and potential service areas
- Establish whether services supply is meeting community needs
- Map flow of clients within various community services
- Determine areas in special need of outreach
- Better identify possible locations for new service branches
- Help with fundraising efforts
- Monitor emerging trends
- To plan routes
- To identify transportation and accessibility issues at specific service areas
- To map geographic distribution of various health and social problems
- To map the location of hazardous-dangerous-toxic sites
- Make an agency's services more attractive and useful to clients
- Open possibility for researchers to study smaller areas and aggregate data to create new units of analysis

One student group participating in the GIS project identified eight of the applications suggested by Queralt and Witte as applicable to their project and added an additional one. According to Norris, Ridel, Scott and Woods (1999), GIS would allow their agency to:

- Visually identify important administrative, policy, and practice issues

PROJECT DEVELOPMENT

With the idea of linkages in mind, of tying together the academic experience of the classroom with the practical experience of the field placement, a funding proposal was developed. It yielded six laptop computers, the necessary GIS software, and a large format (11″ × 17″) color printer. Beyond the tasks of recruitment and selection of participating agencies and students, selection and acquisition of equipment and software, and training of students and development of their research projects, we had no clear plan as to how this project would develop.

Recruiting Agencies

During the summer, letters were sent to the field instructors at the 84 field placement sites then associated with Tulane. The letters described the project and included a copy of an article reporting on a GIS project funded by the Robert Wood Johnson Foundation (Larkin, 1997). Stamped, pre-addressed return envelopes and a reply form were included. Forty-eight replies were received, with 8 indicating definite interest, 16 possibles, and 24 who said they had no interest. Follow-up contacts were made with those that expressed possible interest and 4 were added to the definite interest list.

Recruiting Students

Several weeks after the beginning of the fall semester and the entry of the new MSW class, posters were put up around the school describing the "Bridging" project ("Bridging the Gap Between Research and the Field Practicum") and advising that there would be a meeting for those interested. Sixteen students attended. Using a LCD projector, a PowerPoint presentation about GIS and the "Bridging" project was given, then the GIS program demonstrated. Eight students indicated an interest in participating in the project. It was explained that there were six slots and selection would depend on field assignments, which were made in late October. The criteria would be whether the placement site was one that had indicated a willingness to participate in the program. If the six slots were not filled using that criteria, the student placement sites would be contacted and an effort would be made to recruit the agency's participation. As it was, there was a match between five students and their field placement sites. The other site was one that had not responded to the initial letter, but when contacted, readily indicated an interest in participating.

At an orientation meeting just before the end of the fall semester, participants were issued their laptop computers. There was further discussion of how the GIS project might integrate with their research project, they were checked out on the computers, and provided with a copy of "Mapping Your Community: Using Geographic Information to Strengthen Community Initiatives" (Dept. of Housing & Urban Development, 1997), which was to serve as an introduction to the ways the technology could be used.

Training

Beginning in the spring semester, there was a series of 45-minute, lunchtime meetings where basic skills were demonstrated using an LCD projector. Community 2020 (the software used in the project) provides a seven chapter training manual on its web-site and that served as the framework for the lessons. The skills developed in a chapter were demonstrated, students were provided with a copy of the individual chapter covered, and asked to work through it during the week. At the next session, any questions or problems were addressed and a new topic introduced. The goal of these sessions at this stage was to provide participants with enough understanding of the GIS technology for them to be able to develop (though not necessarily complete) a project at their field site.

As might be anticipated, student computer skill levels varied, as did the rate at which they became comfortable with the GIS technology. Their computer proficiency at the beginning of the program ranged from high to low, though all had some basic computer skills. None had any previous experience with GIS technology. After four sessions, most students felt they had sufficient understanding of the program to begin developing their projects. This led to the decision to terminate the group training and work with students individually on an as-needed basis, with the possibility of more group sessions at a later date. There was much variation in how students' skill levels developed after these classes. One participant developed sufficient expertise to obtain a part-time job working as a research assistant for another professor doing a project using GIS, while another struggled with the technology up to the time the project was completed.

STUDENT PROJECTS

By the end of the spring semester, most students had developed and formalized their research projects. In three situations, visits were paid to student placements to meet with administrators and explain the project and GIS. In the case of two students, extensive one-on-one support was required, but the others developed their projects with a minimal need for support.

Initially, there were six students participating in the project. The usual practice for student research projects is for students to form groups of from 3-6 members. Participants in this project were given the option to work with others or alone. One chose to associate with two others for her project and one of her group members became a participant in the project training. Another formed a group with three other students, all of whom attended the training sessions. The remaining four decided to work on their own. Shortly after the project began, a doctoral student employed with a community agency learned of the project and asked if she could participate. After several months, changes at her agency made participation problematic and she dropped from the program, but her project is included in Table 1. At peak, there were eleven students participating in GIS training and seven projects underway. Table 1 provides a sense of the nature of the projects developed. The significance of GIS varies, with it being an essential component in some cases and a minor add-in in one. Given that the research focus for students was not on GIS, but doing research that would help an agency solve a problem, this was congruent with the project goal of increasing integration of the curriculum.

Students were advised that it was their responsibility to negotiate a project with their agency. While it had to comply with the research sequence requirements for holistic research projects, what they did was their decision. As mentioned, it was emphasized that the focus of their projects should not be GIS, but rather, meeting some real information need of their placement agency. However, several participants became interested in the problem of introducing information technology into the agency setting and asked if they could shift the focus to an examination of that process. In those cases, it was agreed that while they would produce "deliverables" for the agency, their research would take the form of a case study of the introduction of GIS.

PRELIMINARY CONCLUSIONS

This project began with three underlying concerns that coalesced into the goal of training social work students to use GIS technology. In

TABLE 1. Student GIS Projects

PROJECT TITLE	AGENCY TYPE	GOAL OF PROJECT	ROLE OF GIS	RESULTS
Intergeneration Programming at Kingsley House: A Formative Evaluation	A neighborhood-based agency offering a comprehensive range of services	• Formative program evaluation • Demonstrate need for intergenerational programming by mapping area population and existing services	Visualize location of served & unserved clients; availability of resources	No maps were produced. Project emphasis shifted to program evaluation
GIS and Community Analysis	A clinical agency offering services community-wide; moving into community building efforts	• Inform agency planners of perceptions of community problems and needed services vs. actual situation	Create maps that display actual incidence of a range of community problems	Maps produced; student also did case study of efforts to introduce GIS
GIS Software and Social Service Agencies: Making GIS Useful	A community-wide counseling agency	• Case study of introduction of technology • Identify underserved areas	Produce maps to show client base demographics; service area	Student withdrew from MSW program because of illness
An Organizational Analysis of Trinity Counseling and Training Center	A neighborhood-based counseling agency	• Survey agency board members, sponsors and staff to determine perceptions as to agency clientele • Compare with actual demographics	Produce maps to show client base demographics; service area	Maps produced
A Study of Information Needs for a Social Work Agency	A community-wide crisis intervention agency focused on needs of children	• Convert existing database into visual form that can be used for program analysis and development • Identify underserved areas	Produce maps to show client base demographics; service area	Agency unable to provide data; student did case study of efforts to introduce GIS
Development of a GIS-based Routing System for Delivery of Meals to the Home-bound	A community-wide HIV/AIDS information and service agency	• Convert existing manual (paper & pencil) routing system to a computer based one	Produce delivery maps and driving instructions for use by volunteers who change on a frequent basis	Agency director quit; project "put on hold" pending hiring of new director
Utilizing GIS to Identify Gaps in Child Care Services	A neighborhood-based agency offering a comprehensive range of services	• Determine areas of greatest need to fill gaps in child care services • Develop employment opportunities for certified clients • Case study of introduction of technology	Produce maps that can be used for planning purposes	Extensive set of maps produced for agency; case study done by students

developing an instructional approach, a number of decisions were made based on assumptions about how best to approach that goal. The experience of the student participants did much to test those assumptions.

Introduction of Information Technology into the Social Work Curriculum

A scarcity of resources–primarily of time and faculty expertise–made formal classroom instruction in GIS technology impractical. However, sufficient time was found on weekends or during lunch breaks to introduce students to the technology. While those with little computer experience had some anxiety about learning to use the technology, from the student project reports and exit interviews, it is clear that mastery of the GIS software was not a significant concern. The assurance that they had a "tech support" person in the project leader was a factor in this. But the major factor was that the primary concern of the students was not "How do we use this software?" but "What can we do with it?"

Because students were charged with developing a research project using GIS, they had to understand its potential. It was anticipated that the process of learning the software would give them that understanding, but that was an error. For all but one student, who began the project with a high level of computer proficiency, there was not enough time to learn the software, relate it to the needs of their field setting, and negotiate a project with the placement agency. In all but two cases, educating the placement agency about the technology proved to be a major project task. If it had been possible to provide students with a portfolio of "real" examples of how GIS could be used, the project development process might have been simplified considerably, but we were not equipped to do that.

For present purposes, one of the questions raised initially–whether to train students to use applications or to apply them–has been resolved. We will continue to identify early adapters among students and provide them with an opportunity to engage technology directly. Weil, Rosen, and Wugalter (1990), who identified "early adapters" as comprising 10%-15% of the population, suggested they were the ideal leaders in the introduction of technology in the agency setting, and the same may hold true in the academic setting. If given a lead role, their impact can be magnified by their influence on the "hesitant," the

50%-60% of the population who are ambivalent about technology. "Hesitants," if they can be shown that technology can help them, can be as enthusiastic as the "early adapters." Thus, the efforts of "early adapters" can encourage the "hesitants." That is just what happened in this project, where the initial six participants in the project recruited four more.

Increase Integration of the Curriculum

Just as human service agencies are seeking to do more with less by increasing efficiencies, so must social work education. By identifying areas where instruction can be integrated, efforts can be leveraged. To that end, we have begun identifying placement sites that offer research opportunities. One step was for students participating in the GIS project to present their work at the annual orientation for field placement instructors. The goal was to make field instructors more conscious of the possibilities for student research at their agency. At the same time, consideration is being given to modification of the expectations for formal research projects, by allowing a "professional project." While the goal of providing students with a holistic research experience remains unchanged, a broader sense of what is possible will be encouraged.

Introduce GIS Technology into the Social Work/ Human Service Community

As mentioned previously, there are numerous issues involved in the introduction of information technology in the agency setting. A very basic one is awareness of the value of information technology to the profession. The hope had been that students could educate the agency about the technology and that was successful to some extent. In two cases, the agency leadership became interested in the project at an early stage, was supportive throughout, and has begun to explore further uses of GIS. However, in the other, promised support failed to materialize. In future efforts, a formalized agency commitment to participate will be sought. Our experience of the need for strong, top-level involvement supports the conclusion of Phillips and Berman (1995) that a "sponsor" is necessary to successfully introduce information technology into the social work agency (p. 111).

Once the project was underway, it also became apparent that some agencies lacked an understanding of basic information technology "good practices." Students commented on the extent and number of the errors they found in the agency records they were importing into the GIS database. In one case, all of the agency electronic records were archived in a data format that was unintelligible to the programs we were using, and since the person who had created them had left the agency, they were unavailable.

FUTURE STEPS

Through these projects, we hoped to learn more about introducing information technology into the curriculum. This effort has given us the outlines of a model that we hope to develop further in a project involving not only students, but also faculty and agency field instructors. By beginning with those who are interested, giving them a sense of the possibilities of the technology, and the freedom to identify additional ways technology can be of value to social work, it may be possible to meet the concerns that stimulated this project.

REFERENCES

Audet, R.H. & Abegg, G.L. (1996). Geographic information systems: Implications for problem solving. *Journal of Research in Science Teaching, 33 (1)*, 21-45.

Cnaan, R. (1988). Computer illiteracy and human services. *New Technology in Human Services, 4(1)*, 3-8.

Department of Housing and Urban Development (1997). *Mapping your community: Using geographic information to strengthen community initiatives*. Washington, DC: Author. HUD-1092-CPD

Drummond, W.J. (1995). Address matching: GIS technology for mapping human activity patterns. *Journal of the American Planning Association, 61(2)*, 240-251.

England, S., Rivers, L., & Watkins, R. (1999). [Survey of deans and directors of graduate schools of social work regarding distributed and technology-enhanced learning]. Unpublished raw data.

Finn, J. & Lavitt, M. (1995). A survey of information-technology related curriculum in undergraduate social work programs. *The Journal of Baccalaureate Social Work, 1(1)*, 39-53.

Graves, W.H. (1999). On online learning. *Online Learning Resource Kit Vol. 2*. [CD-ROM]. Microsoft Corporation. (available at http://www.microsoft.com/education/hed/online/)

Hernandez, S.H., & Leung, P. (1990). Implementing a social work curriculum on information technology. *Computers in Human Services 7(1-2)*, 113-125.

Hoefer, R.A, Hoefer, R.M., & Tobias, R. (1994). Geographic information systems and human services. *Journal of Community Practice, 1* (3), 113-128.

Larkin, H. (1997). Would you like me to draw a map? *Advances: The Quarterly Newsletter of the Robert Wood Johnson Foundation.* Available on-line *http://www.rwjf.org/library/97-3-2.htm* (accessed 28 July 1999)

Mitchell, A. (1998). *Zeroing in: Geographic information systems at work in the community.* Redlands, CA: Environmental Systems Research Institute.

Norris, W., Ridel, S., Scott, K., & Woods, S. (1999). Utilizing GIS to identify child care service gaps. Unpublished manuscript, Tulane Graduate School of Social Work at New Orleans.

Nurius, P.J., Hooyman, N., & Nicoll, A.E. (1988). The changing face of computer utilization in social work settings. *Journal of Social Work Education, 23(2),* 186-197.

Nurius, P.J., & Nicoll, A.E. (1989). Computer literacy preparation: Conundrums and opportunities for the social work educator. *Journal of Teaching in Social Work, 3(20),* 65-81.

Phillips, D., & Berman, Y. (1995). *Human services in the age of new technology: Harmonizing social work and computerization.* Aldershot, Eng.: Avebury.

Queralt, M., & Witte, A.D. (1998). A map for you? Geographic information systems in the social services. *Social Work, 43(5),* 455-469.

Trabin, T. (Ed.) (1996). *The computerization of behavioral healthcare: How to enhance clinical practice, management, and communications.* San Francisco: Jossey-Bass.

Turkle, S. (1997a). Seeing through computers: Education in a culture of simulation. *The American Prospect, 31 (March-April 1997),* 76-82. Available on-line *http://epn.org/prospect/31/31turkfs.html* (accessed 29 July 1999).

Turkle, S. (1997b). *The future of reading in the age of simulation.* Presentation made at Educom Conference, 1997. Available on-line *http://www.educause.edu/conference/e97/turkle.ram* (accessed 29 July 1999).

Van Lieshout, H., & Roosenboon, P. (1995). From teaching computer technology to social informatics. *New Technology in the Human Services, 8(2),* 6-10.

Wier, R., & Robertson, J. (1998). Teaching geographic information systems for social work applications. *Journal of Social Work Education, 34(1),* 81-96.

APPENDIX A
UNDERSTANDING GIS TECHNOLOGY

HOW IT WORKS

GIS technology makes it easy to produce maps: pin maps, dot-density maps, color-coded maps, scaled-symbol maps, and maps with integrated pie and bar charts. (See Appendix A for a discussion of how GIS technology works.) But to understand how it works, there are a few terms that must be understood.

Layers

The first is that the map one sees is composed of many "layers," each representing some type of geographic feature. When these layers are joined together, a map is created. Layers can represent one of three things: points, lines, and areas. Points may be cities, buildings, addresses, or any other type of discrete visual data. Lines can be things like streets or highways, railroads, rivers, or any other type of continuous visual data. Areas represent contiguous features, such as the position of a city or county, a census tract or block, or a neighborhood.

Themes

Another term one must understand is "theme." This is a method of illustrating the data that goes with a map layer. The data associated with a layer can be represented in different ways. Map "themes" use color, patterns, and symbols to illustrate map features.

Data Sources

The data itself can come from many different sources, though there are three general categories: (1) the census, (2) administrative or agency records, and (3) special surveys. Most GIS packages come with some subset of the 1990 census data (Community 2020, used in this project, includes 647 variables, broken down to census block level), as well as projected data (Community 2020 includes projections for 1997, 2002, and 2007 covering 108 variables down to the census block level). The software makes it possible to associate data (at individual or aggregated levels) with particular layers. Additional data can be added and integrated with that already in the system, expanding its capability to create information.

Geocoding

This feature allows the creation of a layer containing a single geographic point for a single record. The resulting layer can then be used to show where people live, events occur, or building or facilities are located. For example, a separately created database containing the addresses of service recipients can automatically be plotted on a map, providing a visual picture of where clients are coming from.

Routing

This feature combines the geocoding feature with information in an underlying street database to calculate routes. Using information in the system, it calculates distance and time between points, identifies the most efficient routes for travel, and produces a map showing that route and a printout of driving directions.

Making Maps

The maps produced by GIS technology consist of a number of layers of visual features. Associated with each layer is a database file, which contains the data necessary for the software to create the layer. It is possible to view and work with the data file, which means one can change–either by adding, deleting, or editing–the geographic features that appear in the map. At its most basic, map-making is simply a matter of selecting the layers one wishes to see and then customizing the appearance of the map. Beyond that, there are a great many tools that can facilitate the transformation of data into information.

SOFTWARE SELECTION CRITERIA

The basic criteria to be used in selecting software were unclear at the beginning of the project, but emerged as software evaluation proceeded (see Table 2 for software products that were evaluated). They became, in order of priority, ease of use, functionality, and cost.

Ease of Use

As might be anticipated, there is wide variability in their complexity. One of the major developers, ESRI, produces over half a dozen different systems. For our purposes, a system of great sophistication was not necessary. What was necessary was a system that could be easily learned by students (and agency personnel) with widely varying levels of computer skills. For students in the project, that learning would have to occur on their own or in meetings outside of regular class time. Consequently, the system had to be one that could be used without a steep learning curve.

Functions

While the literature provides insight into how GIS technology can be applied to meet information needs in the human services, the emphasis is on the end products of the technology. To decide if a package would be suitable, a clearer sense of the functions and tools needed to produce those end products was necessary. Eventually, a list of possible functions desired was developed, based primarily on examples of applications provided by Mitchell (1998) in "Zeroing In: Geographic Information Systems at Work in the Community." The software selected would have to let the user:

- Find the features of a location and give information about them
- Map characteristics of a neighborhood, town, or city
- Find a location
- Create boundaries
- Get information about people and things in a specific area
- Find the "right" site
- Develop a routing system
- Measure time and distance
- Map complex networks
- Allow easy addition of new data to create new information
- Look for patterns
- Look for trends
- Support planing for future needs on basis of demographic projections

Cost

To allow for software evaluation, a substantial sum was allocated for software in the project budget, so this was not a major consideration. However, as a project concern was to facilitate the introduction of GIS into the agency setting, cost would be a factor. The software would have to be one that an agency with a limited budget for technology might afford.

SOFTWARE PRODUCTS EVALUATED

There are a considerable number of GIS software packages available. The Internet proved to be the most helpful source of information on this technology. Internet research was done and three packages were purchased for evaluation. These were ArcView GIS, produced by ESRI (Environmental Systems Research Institute), Manifold, produced by Manifold Systems, and Community 2020, produced for the Department of Housing and Urban Development by Caliper Corporation. Subsequent to beginning of the project, Microsoft announced it would be offering a mapping product to be called MapPoint 2000. While it appeared too late to be used, a copy was obtained and evaluated on the possibility it might be used later.

The product selected, Community 2020, was developed by HUD to be used by community groups and individuals without extensive technical background. Consequently, it is relatively easy to learn to use. It has geocoding capability (something that is an expensive add-on for other packages), a large data set, and a fairly large set of demographic projections. In addition, it comes with an extensive library of pre-designed maps that can be easily adapted for almost any purpose. That, coupled with its relatively low cost, made it the best suited according to the criteria used.

THE HARDWARE

How programs actually work is a function of individual computer systems, the applications running, and individual operating styles. The package we decided to use–Community 2020–operates on a Pentium PC with 12MB of RAM and a CD-ROM drive (though all necessary

TABLE 2. Products Evaluated

PRODUCT	EASE OF USE	FUNCTIONS	COST
Manifold	A sophisticated package with a steep learning curve. On-line documentation and a minimal tutorial	No geocoding capability, but a broad range of analytic tools; strong mapmaking toolset	$82 (now $145)
ArcView	Moderate learning curve; good documentation & tutorial	Capable of producing sophisticated maps; Has all functions, but geocoding is an add-in	Basic package about $250; geocoding add-in about $500 (academic version)
MapPoint 2000	Moderate learning curve; good on-line help; integrated with Microsoft Office	Minimal functions; not a lot of flexibility in maps that can be produced; small underlying data set	$110
Community 2020	Moderate learning curve; excellent documentation & tutorials; large library of maps that can easily be adapted	Can perform all required functions; includes geocoding functions	$225 for a regional version (US divided into 4 regions)

data can be loaded onto a hard drive). We purchased Compaq Armada 1500 laptop computers equipped with Pentium 166 MHz processors, 32 MB of RAM and 4.3 gig hard drives. We also equipped them with network cards and Microsoft Office Professional.

An LCD projector was used to demonstrate applications in the first and second rounds of training sessions. The second round was held in a conference room with a table wired for network connectivity. This enabled participants to easily share files that had been developed (some were too large to send by e-mail). It also made it possible for them to print to the large format color printer, which was configured for network operation.

APPENDIX B
GIS RESOURCES

Department of Housing and Urban Development (1997). *Mapping Your Community: Using Geographic Information to Strengthen Community Initiatives.* An excellent introduction to the use of GIS describing 17 projects in five cities. It is available free by calling HUD Community Connections at 1-800-998-9999. Ask for the Community 2020 Order Desk to request a copy.

Department of Housing and Urban Development (*http://www.hud.gov/cpd/2020soft.html*) (accessed 29 July 1999).

Manufacturers of Evaluated Software

Caliper Corporation–(*http:////zinfandel.caliper.com/Default.htm*) (accessed 29 July 1999).

ESRI–*http://www.esri.com/index.html* (accessed 29 July 1999).

Manifold Systems–*http://www.manifold.net/* (accessed 29 July 1999).

Microsoft MapPoint 2000–*http://www.microsoft.com/office/mappoint/default.htm* (accessed 29 July 1999).

Databases and Metasites

Geographic Information Systems–*http://www.ummu.umich.edu/library/SUBJECTGUIDES/GIS/GISNR.html* (accessed 29 July 1999).

Robert E. Kennedy Library GIS database–*http://www.lib.calpoly.edu/research/all_databases/gis/gis.html* (accessed 29 July 1999).

GISLinx™–*http://www.gislinx.com/* (accessed 29 July 1999).

The GISPortal–*http://www.gisportal.com/* (accessed 29 July 1999).

From this experience, we can conclude that the introduction of information technology can occur by what Graves (1999) calls "Random Acts of Learning." Before an integrated institutional effort can be developed, a number of such "Acts" will have to occur.

Information Technology and Oppressed Populations: Integration or Isolation?

Julie E. Miller-Cribbs

SUMMARY. Recent research has documented the growing gap between those who have access to information technology and those who do not. Reviewing available literature regarding the lack of access to computers and technology by oppressed groups, this paper discusses problems inherent in ignoring this issue in social work education and practice. Finally, some of the promising interventions currently used to address problems of access are outlined and recommendations for social workers are highlighted. *[Article copies available for a fee from The Haworth Document Delivery Service: 1-800-342-9678. E-mail address: <getinfo@haworthpressinc.com> Website: <http://www.HaworthPress.com> © 2001 by The Haworth Press, Inc. All rights reserved.]*

KEYWORDS. Digital divide, access issues, social work response

Use of information technology (IT) is skyrocketing as more individuals each day utilize e-mail and the world-wide-web (WWW). Social workers, in particular, are using IT in education, practice, and research. Social work sites such as the New Social Worker Magazine, Social Work Cafe, and the Social Work Access Network (SWAN) are accessed by a large number of visitors on a daily basis (Grant & Grobman, 1998).

Julie E. Miller-Cribbs, PhD, is with the College of Social Work, University of South Carolina, Columbia, SC 29208.

[Haworth co-indexing entry note]: "Information Technology and Oppressed Populations: Integration or Isolation?" Miller-Cribbs, Julie E. Co-published simultaneously in *Journal of Technology in Human Services* (The Haworth Press, Inc.) Vol. 18, No. 1/2, 2001, pp. 155-171; and: *Using Technology in Human Services Education: Going the Distance* (ed: Goutham M. Menon, and Nancy K. Brown) The Haworth Press, Inc., 2001, pp. 155-171. Single or multiple copies of this article are available for a fee from The Haworth Document Delivery Service [1-800-342-9678, 9:00 a.m. - 5:00 p.m. (EST). E-mail address: getinfo@haworthpressinc.com].

It is easy to become enamored by IT, its speed, user-friendly nature and provision of current information. It is certainly a valuable social work tool. However, before becoming blinded by the flashes of information on the screen, social workers must remember that resources are only valuable if people can access them. Social work must also concern itself with the widening gap between the information rich and the information poor and pinpoint ways to increase access to oppressed populations. If not, there is risk of isolating disadvantaged populations further.

The goal of this paper is to review issues of access as they relate to oppressed populations. It will discuss the question, *how do social workers use IT and does this use benefit oppressed populations*? By providing a review of the available literature regarding access to information technology by oppressed groups, it will discuss the problems inherent in ignoring this issue in social work. Finally, it will review some of the promising interventions and techniques currently used to address problems of access, explore potential sources of funding for creative and useful interventions using IT, and provide recommendations for social work practice and education.

HOW SOCIAL WORKERS ARE USING INFORMATION TECHNOLOGY

Education. Students are often first exposed to information technology in school and such exposure early in their educational careers is critical to the development of skills that can be translated into practice. In fact, a recent survey of on-line social workers found that 37.7% learned about information technologies in a college or university setting (Marlowe-Carr, 1997). Innovations in distance education using interactive video are utilized in many schools of social work (Foster & Rehner, 1998; Freddolino, 1998; CSWE, 1995; Patchner, Petracchi & Wise, 1998). In addition, interactive videodisc programming is used to simulate social work skills to students. Students are able to practice social work skills with "a touch screen that permits self-paced, self-guided instruction" (Wodarski, Bricourt & Smokowski, 1996).

Many academic departments and professors across disciplines utilize information technology (World Lecture Hall, 1999) and the field of social work is no exception. Students, faculty and staff use electronic mail widely in schools of social work. Social work students access electronic resources such as the Internet or on-line library resources for use in their class assignments (Giffords, 1998). Departments often post important information relevant to students, provide students with links related to their field and provide faculty information. Many also publish their course catalogs and syllabi on line. Many professors also take advantage of online resources in their coursework, including interactive syllabi, suggested links, online discussion groups, or web page projects (see Raymond, Ginsberg & Gohagan, 1998; Coe & Menon, 1999).

Practice. It has been estimated that hundreds of social work related web pages are added to the WWW everyday (Yaffe & Gotthoffer, 1999). Social work practitioners use the Internet to obtain resources for clients, gain information about particular client populations and issues, as well as find support and practice techniques. Advocacy and fundraising is also conducted online by social workers (Grant & Grobman, 1998). Many agencies use the web extensively for policy practice, advocacy and information (Quiero-Tajalli, McNutt & Campbell, 1999). Increasingly information technology has a major role in the policy practice arena and the use of e-mail, web sites, video-teleconferencing, fax, and conference calls are tools of an "emergent electronic advocacy" with which social workers must become involved (Fitzgerald & McNutt, 1997). Information technology is also being used in community development. In response to isolation and lack of support that often goes along with community work, the Cleveland Community Development Corporation Network (CDC Network) developed a network of practitioners who work in community development. The CDC Network uses information technology in an attempt to remove many of the barriers to communication that community workers often face, increase workers' abilities to access relevant information, and to increase support and decrease isolation among community workers (CDC Network, 1999).

The use of information technology also has the ability to decrease the isolation of both social workers and clients in isolated settings. Electronic mail has been used to communicate with homebound or isolated clients such as residents in rural areas as well as elderly clients, disabled individuals and caregivers (Kelly, 1997; Finn, 1997). By providing access to electronic mail and discussion groups, IT has also helped social workers in rural settings, particularly by decreasing levels of isolation.

Social workers also use e-mail to facilitate e-mail support groups and, in Illinois, the Department of Children and Family Services receives some child abuse reports by e-mail (Grant & Grobman, 1998). Such technology-based approaches, sometimes referred to as cybertherapy, have captured the attention of social workers in direct practice and some practice guidelines have been developed (Schopler, Abell, & Galinsky, 1998). Social workers also participate in e-mail or discussion groups where particular practice issues or problems are addressed (Giffords, 1998; Marlowe-Carr, 1997). Finally, some social workers and social work agencies advertise their services on the Internet. Such exposure educates potential clients about the nature of social work and social work services.

OPPRESSED POPULATIONS AND ACCESS TO IT

Just as social work is concerned with inequities in the distribution of society's resources, social work must also concern itself with the phenomenon known as the 'digital divide.' Gaps between the information rich and the information poor continue to expand, thus the information superhighway may actually be more similar to a "limited access toll road" (Stoecker & Stuber, 1997, p.40). Research indicates that discrepancies between certain groups continue to prevail and expand in terms of computer use. Inequities in access based on income, education, race and ethnicity, age, gender, family structure, geographic location, and disability status prevail (Anderson et al., 1995; Benton Foundation, 1998; NTIA, 1998). Groups with the least access to IT are the rural poor, rural and central city minorities, female-headed households and young rural and central city low-income households (NTIA, 1998; Anderson et al., 1995). Interestingly, even within the field of social work the digital divide can be noted, as higher salaried, white, and male social workers access the Internet with the most frequency (Marlowe-Carr, 1999).

Access to computers and information technology is a critical social work issue. Household income and education are strongly correlated with computer use as people with higher income and education have more access to computers, e-mail and information available on the WWW (Coley, Cradler & Engel, 1997; Novak & Hoffman, 1998). It is also important to consider that, unlike the telephone, computer use requires at minimum, *literacy* (Attewell, 1994; Anderson & Bikson,

1998). However, in addition to literacy, the Internet also requires computer-related skills that enable individuals to utilize software. Because this new technology is more complicated, universal access to information technology such as e-mail is a more complex and serious issue (Attewell, 1994; Anderson et al., 1995). Education is essential in such an endeavor, as research has shown that higher levels of education correspond to an increased likelihood of work computer use (Novak & Hoffman, 1998). In an analysis of online content, the Children's Partnership (2000) indicated four main content-related barriers for underserved populations: lack of local information, literacy barriers, language barriers, and lack of cultural diversity.

Populations without adequate access to IT are those with which social work has a vested interest. Racial and ethnic minorities have less access to computers than whites (Novak & Hoffman, 1998; Quiero-Tajalli, McNutt & Campbell, 1999). Individuals between the ages of 35-44 are the most likely to own computers, therefore age also impacts access to IT, with both age extremes, the very young and old, having the least access to computers and the Internet (Benton Foundation, 1998; NTIA, 1995; Finn, 1997). In addition, although the gap between male and female users of computers has lessened in recent years, female-headed households have the lowest levels of use (NTIA, 1995). In fact, single parent families also report lower levels of computer use than two parent families. Individuals with disabilities also have low rates of computer access largely due to the expense of equipment that enables individuals with disabilities to utilize IT (Neuman, 1991). Further, it has been argued that in some cases, online learning creates more barriers for students with disabilities than opportunities (Nussbaum, 2000). This is particularly problematic as assistive technologies have enormous potential for helping children with special needs (U.S. Department of Education, 1996).

Although some progress has been made since Clinton announced his technology plan (American's Technology Literacy Challenge, 1996), poor students, schools and communities still do not have equitable access to information technology (Benton Foundation, 1998; NCES, 1999; U.S. Department of Education, 1996; Glennan & Melmed, 1996). Overall public schools lag far behind in terms of their access to new technologies and poor minority students and high poverty schools have even fewer computers and modems than affluent students and schools (Furger, 1999; U.S. Department of Education, 1996; NCES,

1999). This is worrisome as poor, minority students are also less likely to have access to computers in their homes (NCES, 1999).

However, the presence of a computer alone does not guarantee that students will gain the necessary skills to use them. Although the use of computers in education has been linked with the development of higher order thinking skills, disadvantaged children are less likely to be exposed to the kind of training that would enable them to develop these skills. Acquisition of such analytical skills on the part of students requires that educators have the requisite skills to facilitate computer-based learning. Unfortunately, research indicates that many poor minority students use computers for drills or games where higher order skills are not developed (Neuman, 1991; Furger, 1999; Glennan & Melmed, 1996; U.S. Department of Education, 1996). Thus, "economically disadvantaged students, who often use the computer for remediation and basic skills, learn to do what the computer tells them, while more affluent students, who use it to learn programming and tool applications, learn to tell the computer what to do" (Neuman, 1991, p. 2). Students who develop analytical skills and learn to control the computers will also have a greater chance at controlling their own destinies.

Finally, because individuals who are not disadvantaged dominate the development and use of IT, the issue of diversity arises. Most of the web sites on the WWW are designed by young white males and often do not capture the interests or cultures of a diverse society (Quiero-Tajalli et al., 1999). Although generalized cultural sites for certain ethnic and racial groups are appearing on the WWW, overall there is not much cultural information on the local level (Children's Partnership, 2000). Sites that provide for opportunities to explore and develop culture, that advertise or inform people of local ethnic and cultural events and interests, and that provide other important and relevant local information geared to specific racial and ethnic groups (health, housing, jobs) are not widely available (Children's Partnership, 2000). In all, it is no wonder that disenfranchised individuals are not easily convinced of the benefits of technology. A report from the Benton Foundation (1998) notes that,

> Many low income people themselves are skeptical about the value of digital technologies. This isn't surprising, since poor people have little exposure to the new technologies and their

experiences with previous technologies may not have been as positive as middle-class policy makers might assume. (p. 2)

A recent study found that relatively more African American and Hispanics had no knowledge of the WWW and over half of those individuals who reported they had not heard of the WWW had incomes below $25,000 (Benton Foundation, 1998). The reality is that part of being poor and disadvantaged is being disconnected from society's resources, including information technology. Even though it may seem to most Americans that cyberculture is a part of everyday life, the reality is that many Americans are not even aware of the WWW and how it relates to their lives.

DANGERS INHERENT IN CONTINUED DISPARITIES IN ACCESS TO IT

Some of the benefits of utilizing IT in social work have been previously discussed. However, there are also benefits provided to individuals and communities who have access to IT. Anderson et al. (1995) document the benefits of access to IT in a recent RAND report. They note that electronic networks have the potential to improve communication–including community building and social integration, improve access to information, facilitate the restructuring of non-profit and community based organizations, and promote efficacy and increased responsiveness of public institutions. Without a doubt, IT has tremendous potential in the field of social work.

However, social workers must also ensure that inequities in access to IT are addressed. One of the most pressing concerns may be that the Internet is rapidly becoming the only location where critical information, particularly government information, is made available to the public (Stoecker & Stuber, 1997; Long-Scott, 1995). This has devastating consequences for those without access to information about certain government programs, policies or jobs. Not only will individuals who are information poor lack access to the lists of jobs; they will also lack access to online supports (e-mail, list-serves) that help them succeed in the competitive job market (Stoecker & Stuber, 1997). Anderson and Bikson (1998) note that "digital government, and digital libraries imply that most Americans will have to become Internet literate in the near future just to carry out the day-to-day activities of citizens in a developed society, quite independently of the computer demands made on them by their workplace" (p. 1).

Not only are disadvantaged individuals at risk for losing access to information, but agencies that serve such populations will be at risk of missing critical information as well. Stoecker and Stuber (1997) address this issue particularly as it relates to neighborhood-based organizations (NBOs). They note that NBOs consist of individuals within a certain neighborhood and are small, isolated, and lack financial resources. In addition, members of NBOs frequently do not have efficient access to information that would assist them in understanding the problems in their neighborhood or ideas and resources needed to solve complex neighborhood problems. With the trend toward decentralization, locally based neighborhood groups will continue to struggle to keep up with an increasingly digital world and consequently, communities served by these agencies will suffer (Long-Scott, 1995; Kreig, 1995; Seron & Horrigan, 1997). Although many foresee that public schools and libraries will provide poor communities access to IT, most schools and libraries in low-income communities tend to mirror the gap in resources as opposed to closing it (Benton Foundation, 1998). In fact, "there is a direct link between the wealth of a library's neighborhood and the ability of that library to serve its neighborhood information needs" (Benton, 1998). Historically, there have been some problems with telecommunications providers as well, with companies not providing poor communities with new services (Benton Foundation, 1998; Long-Scott, 1995). In the end, this 'redlining' of IT could have a devastating impact on low-income minority communities, particularly in terms of democratic participation in government and access to critical information (Long-Scott, 1995; Kreig, 1995; Seron & Horrigan, 1997).

Social work must also avoid the redlining of information. Although advertising social work services on the WWW is beneficial for some clients, such use will certainly cream to computer users that at this time, by and large, are not oppressed. Even more dangerous is the provision of certain services on the WWW. For example, recently there has been a proliferation of adoption services on the web. Many of these web sites provide critical information to potential adoptive parents, which often include pictures and summaries of children to be adopted. While this is certainly a valuable resource, social work must not forget the many individuals who do not have access to this vital information.

Cost is also a serious barrier. Equipment is often expensive and complicated. Rural and central city communities often do not have access to lines that would enable to connect them to the WWW, even if they had access to computer equipment. Small, low budget agencies frequently do not have the resources to provide their workers with access to computers or training (Stoecker & Stuber, 1999). For example, in a recent study of 189 Ohio urban neighborhood-based organizations, only three agencies had complete access to the WWW (Stoecker & Stuber, 1999). Much of the software that is developed for social service agencies is expensive and often requires expensive equipment (modems, computers, printers, networks) as well as significant time and money (Oyersman & Benbenishty, 1999; Stiedjer & Stuber, 1999). However, "unless social workers do become involved in the ways in which new technologies are used within organizations, they will fail to influence its impact upon their clients and may further fail to control the way in which computers affect the nature of social work itself in the future" (Sapey, 1997, p. 803).

WHAT IS BEING DONE?

Despite the disparaging reports of inadequate access to information technology among oppressed populations, numerous promising and innovative programs and policies have been developed. The following section highlights the main policies and programs that may be of interest to social workers. In addition, Table 1 highlights links that provide excellent information and resources.

Clinton's 1996 Technology Literacy Challenge committed the federal government to assist every school and library to become wired to the WWW by 2000. This aggressive policy has promoted a great deal of research and programmatic interest. The Telecommunications Act of 1996 also helped to make telecommunications services and technologies available to schools and libraries at reduced rates, commonly known as the E-Rate (Education Rate). As a result, the number of classes connected to the WWW has increased and helped over 30,000 schools and libraries connect to the WWW (NCES, 1999; Furger, 1999). In addition, the act established the Telecommunications Development Fund which is designed to elevate access to capital for small

TABLE 1. Selected List of Organizations Reviewed

Pennsylvania Digital Grassroots	http://L2L.org/DG/about.html
What's Working in Education Benton Foundation	http://www.benton.org/Practice/Edu
National Institute for Technology Planning	http://www.nctp.com/
FCC Disabilities Issues Task Force	http://www.fcc.gov/dtf/
Benton Foundation Universal Access	http://www.benton.org/Policy/Uniserv/uniserv.html
Fostering the Use of Educational Technology: Elements of a National Strategy RAND	http://www.rand.org/publications/MR/MR682/contents.html
VICNET	http://www.vicnet.net.aut
NetAction	http://netaction.org/training
Markle Foundation	http://www.markle.org
RAND	http://www.rand.org
Benton Foundation - Advocacy on the Internet	http://www/benton.org/practice/Best/advoc.html
NTIA	http://www.ntia.gov
CDC Network	http://little.nhlink.net/nhlink/cdc/
Electronic Advocacy in Social Work Practice	http://www.bc.edu/bc_org/avp/gssw/ea_resources.html
Children's Partnership	http://www.childrenspartnership.org

businesses, stimulate new technology development, provide support for universal service, and to promote telecommunications services to underserved populations (Benton Foundation, 1996). Also included in the Telecommunications Act are provisions for increasing access to persons with disabilities. A Disabilities Issues Task Force, under the FCC, also provides information and resources for increasing access to IT for people with disabilities. In addition, the Office of Telecommunications and Information Applications has two programs designed to promote telecommunications and support projects that increase access of undeserved inner city and remote rural minority populations to social service information that is available online. The Department of Education also provides funding for technology innovation challenge grants.

There are several notable organizations who have contributed by increasing knowledge regarding the gaps between the information poor and information rich, highlighting innovative uses of technology, evaluating technology related programs and policy, advocating for technology in schools and communities, and promoting research on universal access to e-mail (Benton Foundation, RAND, U.S. Department of Education, National Center on Education Statistics, NTIA, Markle Foundation, The Children's Partnership) Extensive research reports, conference proceedings, grant information, and examples of technology based reports are available at the web sites of these organizations.

There are several technology based approaches currently used to alleviate a myriad of complex social problems and some are available online. For example, the Benton Foundation (1998) reports on several projects on their "What's Working" website, where best practices for using IT in low-income communities and schools as well as conducting advocacy are listed. Pennsylvania has many innovative programs including Build PEN, which is an organization that installs free donated wiring to schools and training for teachers. Project NEAT assists schools in the Appalachian region obtain connections to the WWW. In addition, Pennsylvania created the Digital Grassroots Initiative that was designed specifically to provide students with technology skills and support teacher training. This teacher training also includes the provision of lesson plans and projects on the WWW. These resources are compiled on a Link-to-Learn web site and are used by teachers for professional development. Digital Grassroots also attempts to help business and organizations set up WWW sites and provide communities with Internet access and community information. Several other organizations offer information and resources for increasing the use of technology in schools (see Benton Foundation, National Center for Technology Planning, RAND, NCES, and U.S. Department of Education). Glennan and Melmed (1996) detail the use and effectiveness of educational technology and highlight the experiences of some schools that have had previous success using educational technology. They also address the challenges of helping schools integrate technology into their classrooms, and conclude with policy recommendations.

Other agencies address how to increase oppressed populations' access to IT as well as how to use IT to improve access to resources. For example, universal e-mail and community-based networks have tremendous potential in low-income communities. Community voice mail programs have been found to be a very useful tool by providing homeless individuals access to a phone number. Other agencies, such as LibertyNet in Philadelphia, attempt to make the WWW available to the entire community. Free technology courses for community groups and individuals are also provided. In Australia, VICNET offers free user directories, HTML training, and support for uploading web sites. In Ohio, the Urban University and Neighborhood Network tries to bring together universities and NBOs to share resources in order to better serve low-income neighborhoods. There is also an emergent literature discussing the benefits of civic networks (see Anderson et al., 1996). In California, East Bay community groups created a collaboration of organizations that support Neighborhood Network Centers in some HUD assisted properties. The Crescent Park Multi-Cultural Family Resource Center "operates 20 workstation computers and provides Internet access, video conferencing and distance learning satellite links" (Weger, 1999).

There is also enormous potential for advocacy on the Internet. In addition, some organizations offer online training for conducting online advocacy such as NetAction, which provides an online course on virtual activism. In addition, McNutt (1999) maintains a very helpful web site entitled "Electronic Advocacy in Social Work Practice." The Benton Foundation also provides examples of organizations providing advocacy on the Internet as well as offering a critique of each site–recognizing both the strengths and weaknesses of each organization's efforts.

CONCLUSIONS AND RECOMMENDATIONS

Ultimately social work strives towards ensuring that individuals have equal access to society's resources. Given the inevitable and important integration of IT into the field of social work, social workers must take the lead in finding ways to create increased access to oppressed populations. The following are some general recommendations for social workers.

Advocate for policy that ensures equitable access to information technology. Policy that includes universal access to e-mail, increased funding for non-profit community based organizations and public institutions such as libraries are essential elements needed to facilitate equitable access to IT. Recently, legislation has been introduced that threatens the E-Rate for schools and libraries and social workers should advocate for keeping the E-Rate available. Novak and Hoffman (1998) note that minority students need multiple points of access to IT, including in the school, home, and library and public policy should address such discrepancies in access. More recently the city of Oakland, California passed a 1997 resolution that mandates that all new public housing projects have advanced telecommunications services (Hakala, 1998). Currently, Congress is considering the Digital Empowerment Act which would created a one-stop shop for technology education, increase resources for training and school technology, expand e-rate, create an 'e-corps' within the Americorps program, put technology in public housing and create 1,000 new Community Technology Centers. These are just two examples of policies that have potential to dramatically increase access to information technologies and should be of concern to social workers. Although historically social work has not placed emphasis on communications or technology policy, in order to ensure equitable access to information technologies, social work must certainly consider integrating technology policy issues into social work education, research and practice. As Quiero-Tajalli et al. (1999) note, "All social workers must be prepared to take up the cause of social and economic justice in the information age" (p. 15).

Increase the computer skills of social workers and educate social work students regarding the role of IT in social work practice. Increasing students' own efficacy with computer skills–so they take these skills to agencies and to clients–is critical. Many social work clients do not have access to computers and it will be social workers with computer knowledge and skills leading the way and bridging these gaps. Such skills could include the development of innovative programs for use in schools, libraries and other public institutions, web authoring, or electronic advocacy. Social workers can be critical to the development of websites that are culturally relevant, accessible, bilingual and inclusive of important local and community information. Social work students must also be reminded that until universal access is achieved, reliance on IT for practice will inevitably alienate those without access to computers.

Evaluate the role of social work and the use of IT. What does it mean to practice social work electronically? What are the ethical dilemmas in such an endeavor? Certainly social work must design practice guidelines that address technology issues (Schopler et al., 1999) and social workers must know how to use computers (Miller-Cribbs & Chadiha, 1998; Giffords, 1998). As Smith (1999) notes, "if we fail to step back and imagine how our work can be fundamentally transformed, we are at best doomed to shoehorn traditional techniques into the new medium, much like using a video to record slide shows" (p. 31). Further, if social work practice will occur via e-mail or using online groups, certainly guidelines for such activities must be incorporated into the social work code of ethics. Other related fields have addressed these issues and have adopted guidelines for online practice (see, for example: American Psychological Association, 2000; American Counseling Association, 2000). Cwikel and Cnaan (1991) note that it is critical that social workers consider how social work values will be included in the use of advanced technologies and guarantee that the uses of these technologies promote quality social work practice.

Conduct research on IT and social work. Many social workers have already begun to address both the advantages and disadvantages of the use of information technology in the field of social work (Krueger & Stretch, 1997; Miller-Cribbs & Chadiha, 1998) and this is certainly an important debate. Yet, the reality is, while social workers debate the issue, more and more individuals access the Internet each day. Increasingly, social workers and social work agencies take advantage of online support groups, use the Internet for advertisement of services, or use technology for data management and referrals (Giffords, 1998; Belew, 1999; Wellness International Network, 1999). Thus, it is important for social workers to understand how to use technology in the best interest of clients.

Social workers must place themselves within the debate on universal access to IT, its implications for society as a whole and for the profession of social work. Interventions using computer-based techniques must be evaluated and integrated into practice knowledge. Social work must also focus on how to improve access to IT for oppressed populations and how to transform the WWW so that it reflects the diversity of the population.

REFERENCES

American Counseling Association. (April, 2000) Special Message: Ethical Standards for Internet on-line counseling. [WWW document] URL *http://www.counseling.org/gc/cybertx.html*

American Psychological Association. (April 2000). Services by telephone, teleconferencing and Internet. [WWW document] URL *http://apa.org/ethnic/stmnt01.html*

American's Technology Literacy Challenge (February, 1996) [WWW document] URL *http://www.whitehouse.gov/WH/New/edteh/2pager.html*

Anderson, R., & Bikson, T. (1998). Focus on Generic Skills for Information Technology Literacy, RAND Report P-8018. [WWW document] URL *http://www.rand.org/publications/P/P8018*

Anderson, R., Bikson, T., Law, S., & Mitchell, B. (1995). Universal Access to E-mail: Feasibility and Societal Implications, RAND Report MR-650-MI. [WWW document] URL *http://www.rand.org/publications/MR/MR650/*

Attewell, P. (1994). Computer-Related Skills and Social Stratification. Presented at Universal E-mail: Prospects and Implications, RAND, 1994.

Belew, K. (January, 1999) The Complete Social Worker's Guide to Using the Internet in Social Work. [WWW document] URL *http://hadm.sph.sc.eedu.Students/KBelew/csw.htm*

Benton Foundation (1998). Losing ground bit by bit: Low-income communities in the information age. [WWW document] URL *http://www.benton.org/Library/Low-Income/*

Benton Foundation (1996). The telecommunications act of 1996 and the changing landscape of communications. [WWW document] URL *http://www.benton.org/Library/Landscape/landscape.html*

Children's Partnership (2000). Online content for low-income and underserved Americans, The digital divide's new frontier. Santa Monica, CA: The Children's Partnership.

Cleveland Community Development Corporation Network (April, 1999). [WWW document] URL *http://little.nhlink.net/nhlink/cdc/cdc-idx.htm*

Coe, J. & Menon, G. (1999). *Computers and information technology in social work education, training & practice*. NY: The Haworth Press, Inc.

Coley, R., Cradler, J. & Engel, P. (1997). Computers and Classrooms: The Status of Technology in US Schools. ETS Policy Information Center. Princeton, NJ [WWW document] URL *http://www.ets.org/research/pic/compclass/html*

Commission on Accreditation, CSWE (1995). Guidelines for SW Distance Education programming. Alexandria, VA.

Cwikel, J. & Cnaan, R. (1991). Ethical dilemmas in applying second-wave information technology to social work practice. *Social Work 36(2)*, 114-120.

Federal Communications Commission (September, 1998). Telecommunications Act of 1996. [WWW document] URL *http://www.fcc.gov/telecom.html*

Finn, J. (1997). Aging and information technology: The promise and the challenge. *Generations, 21*, 5-6.

Fitzgerald, E. & McNutt, J.G. (1997). Electronic advocacy in policy practice: A framework for teaching technologically based practice. Paper presented at the CSWE Annual Program meeting, Chicago, IL.

Foster, M. & Rehner, T. (1998). Part-Time MSW Distance Education: A Program Evaluation. *Computers in Human Services 14, 2/3*, 9-22

Freddolino, P. (1998). Building on experience: Lessons from a distance education MSW program. *Computers in Human Services 14, (2)*, 339-50.

Furger, R. (September, 1999). Are Wired Schools Failing Our Kids? PC World Online. [WWW document] URL *http://www.pcworld.com:80/share*

Giffords, E. (1998). Social Work on the Internet: An Introduction. *Social Work, 43 (3)*, 243-253.

Glennan, T. & Melmed, A. (1996). Fostering the use of educational technology: Elements of a national strategy. RAND MR-682-OSTP. [WWW document] URL *http://www.rand.org/publications/MR/MR682/contents.html*

Grant, G. & Grobman, L. (1998). *The Social Worker's Internet Handbook*. Harrisburg, PA: White Hat Communications.

Grobman, L. & Grant, G. (1998). *The non-profit Internet handbook*. Harrisburg, PA: White Hat Communications.

Hakala, D. (1998). Sm@rt Reseller *http://www.2dnet.com/sr/business/opportunity/hotel.html*

Heaviside, S., Riggins, T. & Farris, E. (February, 1997). Advanced Telecommunications in US Public Elementary and Secondary Schools, Fall 1996. National Center for Education Statistics NCES 97-944. [WWW document] URL *http://www.nces.ed.gov/pubs/97944.html*

Kelly, K. (1997). Building aging programs with online information technology. *Generations 21*, 15-18.

Kreig, R. (1995). Information technology and low-income, inner city communities. *The Journal of Urban Technology. 3 (1)* Fall.

Krueger, L. & Stretch, J. (1997). Hyper-technology is destroying social work. Paper presented at the National Conference Information Technologies for Social Work Education, Charleston, SC.

Long-Scott, A. (1995) *Access Denied. Outlook, 8 (1)* Summer.

Marlowe-Carr, L. (1997). Social workers on-line: A profile. *Computers in Human Services, 14 (2)*, 59-70.

Miller-Cribbs, J. & Chadiha, L. (1998). Integrating the internet in a human diversity course. *Computers in Human Services, 15 (2/3)*, 97-103.

National Center for Educational Statistics (Feb, 1999). Internet Access in Public Schools and Classrooms: 1994-98 Issue Brief (NCES 99-017) [WWW document] *http://nces.ed.gov/pubs99/1999017.html*

National Telecommunications and Information Administration (NTIA) (1998) Falling Through the Net II: New data on the digital divide. [WWW document] URL *http://www.ntia.doc.gov/ntiahome/net21*

National Telecommunications and Information Administration (NTIA) (1995) Falling Through the Net: A Survey of 'Have Nots' in Rural and Urban America. [WWW document] URL *http://www.ntia.doc.gov/ntiahome/fallingthru.html*

National Telecommunications and Information Administration (NTIA) (1995) Grants and Assistance for Minorities [WWW document] URL *http://www.ntia.doc.gov/otiahome/maassist.html*

Neuman, D. (1991). Technology and Equity. ERIC Digest ED 339400. [WWW document] URL *http://www.ed.gov/databases/ERIC_Digests/ed339400.html*

Novak, T. & Hoffman, D. (February, 1998). Bridging the Digital Divide: The Impact of Race on Computer Access and Internet Use. Project 2000, Vanderbilt University. [WWW document] URL *http://www2000.ogsm.vanderbilt.edu/papers/race/science.html*

Nussbaum, D. (March, 2000). For the disabled, barriers to online study. New York Times on the Web. [WWW document] URL *http://www10.nytimes.com/library/national/040900edlife-oneline-edu.html*

Oyersman, D. & Benbenishty, R. (1997). Developing and implementing the integrated information system for foster care and adoption. *Computers in Human Services, 14 (1)*, 1-20.

Patchner, M., Petracchi, H., & Wise, S. (1998). Outcomes of ITV and Face-to-Face Instruction in a social work research methods course. *Computers in Human Services 14, 2/3* 23-38

Petterson, D., Pullen, L., Evers, E., Champlin, D. & Ralson, T. (1997). An experimental evaluation of HyperCDTX: Multimedia substance abuse treatment education software. *Computers in Human Services, 14 (1)*, 21-38.

Quiero-Tajalli, I., McNutt, J., & Campbell, C. (1999). Electronic advocacy by Latino organizations: Implications for practice and education. Paper presented at the 1999 CSWA Annual Program Meeting, San Francisco, CA.

Raymond, F., Ginsberg, L. & Gohagan, D. (1998). *Information Technologies: Teaching to use, using to teach*. NY: The Haworth Press, Inc.

Sapey, B. (1997). Social work tomorrow: Towards a critical understanding of technology in social work. *British Journal of Social Work, 27 (6)*, 803-814.

Schopler, J., Abell, M. & Galinsky, M. (1998) Technology-Based Groups: A Review and Conceptual Framework for Practice. *Social Work 43 (3)*, 254-267.

Seron, L. & Horrigan, J. (1997). Urban Poverty and Access to Information Technology: A Role for Local Government. *Journal of Urban Technology 4(3)*, 61.

Smith, C. (1999). *Family life pathfinders on the new electronic frontier. 48*, 31-34.

Stoecker, R. & Stuber, A. (1997). Limited access: The information superhighway and Ohio's Neighborhood-Based Organizations. *Computers in Human Services, 14 (2)*, 39-57.

U.S. Department of Education (1997). US Department of education technology innovation challenge grants [WWW document] URL *http://www.ed.gov/Technology/challenge*

U.S. Department of Education (1995). Synthesis of major issues of Secretary's conference on educational technology. [WWW document] URL *http://www.ed.gov/Technology/Plan/MakeHappen/Issue1.html*

Vernon, R. & Lynch, D. (2000). *Social work and the web*. Belmont, CA: Wadsworth.

Weger, B. (1999). Bridging the Digital Divide in the San Francisco bay area. *Neighborhood Network News*. [WWW document] URL *http://www.hud.gov/nnw/nnw-data/NEW-0358.html*

Wellness International Network (3 January, 1999). [WWW document] URL *http://www.wellnessnet.com/a-socialworker-index.htm*

Wodarski, J., Bricourt, J., & Smokowski, P. (1996) Making Interactive Videodisc Computer Simulation Accessible and Practice Relevant. *Journal of Teaching in Social Work 13 1/2*, 15-26

World Lecture Hall (1999). [WWW document] URL *http://www.utexas.edu/world/lecture/*

Yaffe, J. & Gotthoffer, D. (1999). *Quick guide to the internet for social work*. Boston: Allyn & Bacon.

Index

To my family, whose love is boundless and is never avoidant.